Conversion
Course

1991 1

CLINICAL N
AND DIETETIC!

GW00871446

MODERN NURSING SERIES

General Editor
SUSAN E NORMAN, SRN, DN Cert, RNT
Senior Tutor, The Nightingale School, St Thomas's Hospital, London

Consultant Editor
A J HARDING RAINS, MS, FRCS
Regional Dean, British Postgraduate Medical Federation;
formerly Professor of Surgery, Charing Cross Hospital Medical School;
Honorary Consultant Surgeon, Charing Cross Hospital;
Honorary Consultant Surgeon to the Army

This series caters for the needs of a wide range of nursing, medical and ancillary professions.
Some of the titles are given below, but a complete list is available from the Publisher.

General Surgery and the Nurse
R E HORTON

Intensive Care
A K YATES, P J MOORHEAD and A P ADAMS

Taverner's Physiology
DERYCK TAVERNER

Community Health and Social Services
BRIAN DAVIES

Community Child Health
MARION E JEPSON

Textbook of Medicine
L R J HARRISON

Revision Notes on Psychiatry
K T KOSHY

CLINICAL NUTRITION AND DIETETICS FOR NURSES

A W GOODE
MD, FRCS

Assistant Director and Reader in Surgery
The Surgical Unit, The London Hospital

J P HOWARD
SRD

District Dietitian
Hammersmith and Fulham Health Authority

S WOODS
SRN, DipN

Clinical Nutrition Sister
St Mark's Hospital

HODDER AND STOUGHTON
LONDON SYDNEY AUCKLAND TORONTO

British Library Cataloguing in Publication Data

Goode, Anthony
    Clinical nutrition and dietetics for nurses.
    —(Modern nursing series)
    1. Nutrition   2. Nursing
    I. Title   II. Howard, Pat   III. Woods, Suzanne
    IV. Series
    613.2'024613   RT87.N87

    ISBN 0 340 36596 X

First published 1985

Typeset by
Macmillan India Ltd, Bangalore

Printed in Great Britain for Hodder and Stoughton Educational, a division of Hodder and
Stoughton Ltd, Mill Road, Dunton Green, Sevenoaks, Kent. TN13 2YD by
Richard Clay (The Chaucer Press) Ltd, Bungay, Suffolk

Editor's Foreword

Without the adequate provision of food any nation or community declines, is disordered and falls apart. No government or leader dare ignore this first and simple rule or axiom and to do so is to court dismissal or worse. And with the human body inadequate provision of nutrition leads to decline, disorder and falling apart, particularly after injury or operation. But in this case and within the context of medical and nursing practice the failure to observe simple rules ends in the demise of the patient rather than the disgrace of those supposed to be in command. The matter deserves the highest priority amongst the skills we learn and we need a text to keep us properly informed and instructed about every situation. How surprising it is to learn that even in our midst in a well endowed society so many people admitted to hospital are severely under or imperfectly nourished. How sad it is when this state of malnutrition goes unrecognised and uncorrected, say, before operation, or that nutritional decline is not appreciated, measured and corrected during the post operative period or in a post infective illness. Even more regretful is it to observe that those who need assistance with feeding are not fed.

This subject becomes a real exercise on the meaning of 'care', namely to care about what can happen and does happen if . . . , to care about the recognition of nutritional deficiency, to care about skilful, adequate and compassionate restoration. I recommend this book by accomplished, experienced authors for daily use as a good companion by those who believe they care, or who begin to realise that they must take the greatest care to master this fundamental subject.

A J Harding Rains

Preface

The last fifteen years have seen a revolution in patient care with a return to basic principles. An increasing awareness of the importance of nutrition and maintenance of health in the successful management of disease has led to great changes in nursing practice. This book is designed to explain the theoretical background to nutritional care and particular emphasis is placed on the role of the nurse in enteral and parenteral nutrition.

The rapid expansion of knowledge has resulted in uncertainty and some confusion about the principles and daily practice of nutritional support. We believe this integrated approach ranging from basic principles to complex practice will provide a useful understanding of an important contribution to better patient care.

We thank Professor A J Harding Rains for his unfailing support and encouragement. The nursing staff at Charing Cross Hospital have been an invaluable and unfailing source of advice. We thank in particular Miss Kate Smalley, Clinical Nurse Manager, The Surgical Unit, Miss J Isard, The School of Nursing, Mrs M Greatbatch and Mrs M Elwood-Russell. Our thanks also to the Department of Nutrition and Dietetics, Charing Cross, for their help, to Ms Janice Everett and Miss Elizabeth Grant, who typed the manuscript, and Gregory Mason for the illustrations. Susan Devlin and Alison Fisher at Hodder and Stoughton have been invaluable, together with Mr W H Goode who read the proofs.

A W GOODE
J P HOWARD
S WOODS

Contents

General explanation of the text

The various dietary modifications which are commonly encountered have been identified and categorised. This is presented as follows:

1 *Aim* of the particular dietary restriction.

2 An outline of some of the *relevant drugs* which may be prescribed (these are not intended to be exhaustive lists).

3 *Important points* which should *always* be remembered in the context of the described diet.

4 An outline of the *general modifications* which should be made to the hospital menu in order to conform with a specific dietary prescription.

5 *General observations* which may be helpful.

It is important to remember that methods of food service and delivery vary between hospitals – particularly in respect of the way in which meals are actually ordered. Any such local factors should be carefully checked *before* applying the following information.

I
Introduction

'Il faut manger pour vivre – non pas vivre pour manger' (*'One should eat to live – not live to eat'*)   Molière

From the dawn of history, the most pressing human concern has been securing food to satisfy hunger. Proper nutrition is essential for growth, repair after injury and energy production and as such is a fundamental human requirement. For the greater part of recorded time whatever was edible was eaten without any understanding of its nutrient value, taste and satisfaction being the only criteria. In ancient times the more enlightened physicians realised the importance of food. Hippocrates (400 BC), the father of medicine, paid strict attention to the diets of his patients but it is clear from his writing that he had little understanding of the nature of nutrition, believing, for example, that cheese produced flatulence and constipation.

The earliest recorded observations and experiments in nutrition with human subjects are recorded in the Old Testament in the book of Daniel. Daniel asked that he and his Jewish friends of the court of Nebuchadnezzar be excused the ritual of the court. While they were training they lived on vegetables, herbs and water and, of course, were very quickly fitter and leaner than those living well from the King's table. About 200 BC Athaenus, a Greek living in Rome, wrote the earliest recorded cookery book and commentary on foods in relation to health. Although it is of historical interest, it reveals the state of ignorance and credulity of educated and prominent men of the time as, for example, cabbage was extolled as the ideal remedy against the intoxicating effects of wine.

Through the centuries the experience of mankind with good and bad food led reflective men to believe that diet had much to do with health. In the 17th century measurement and observation began when in 1614 Sanctorius recorded the variations in his weight after eating, drinking, sleeping and resting. In the 18th century there were two important scientific studies of nutrition; Lavoisier showed that animals were complex engines which required food to generate body heat, and von Liebig discovered that animals were composed of protein, carbohydrate and fat. In the early 19th century Rubner investigated the relationship between energy consumption and the components of body composition. He and other workers reached the conclusion that body weight is made up of fat and a lean body mass which in turn is composed of muscle, skeleton and viscera. The lean body mass is the active metabolic component of the body and chemical analysis showed that it was rich in nitrogen, potassium and water, unlike fat. In the latter half of the 19th century the importance of electrolytes in the body, particularly potassium and sodium, were recognised and further research prior to the First World War identified other essential dietary components, including vitamins, some trace elements and the essential fatty acids.

Chronic under-nutrition and starvation have been common problems through the ages. Donovan in 1848 described the autopsy findings in the victims of the Irish potato famine. He noticed the total disappearance of the omentum, and the peculiarly thin and transparent condition of the small intestine as well as the marked loss of body fat and skeletal muscle, together with shrinkage of the heart. This showed that many parts of the body are affected by lack of food.

That patients require adequate feeding is an old concept dating to Hippocrates. O'Shaunessy in 1893 reported complex chemical changes in the blood of cholera victims and later cured some patients by the rapid intravenous injection of salt. In 1860 Claud Bernard and in 1863 Hodder gave milk intravenously to cholera patients. By 1900 glucose, a sugar, was infused as a calorie or energy source and in the 1930's fat solutions were developed together with enzymatic hydrolysed protein solutions for intravenous use as a nitrogen source.

The preferred method of delivery of the required nutrients has for many decades been into the gastrointestinal tract. However, the intravenous route is now also available due to the technological advances during the last twenty years in intravenous catheter development for placement into major veins.

From the historical background and from the understanding gained it has become evident that impaired nutrition is a common feature in many disease states. A compromised nutritional status has extensive consequences which may result in an increased mortality rate in wasted patients undergoing major surgery and many more subtle complications such as the failure of wounds to heal, altered drug metabolism, weakness, apathy, depression and an increased inability to resist infection—all of which may add to the time that the patient will be in hospital. Now with modern scientific and technological developments the means are available to correct malnutrition in hospital patients.

2
What Is Good Nutrition?

The study of good nutrition is generating much interest at the present time. The fact that every individual needs 'good nutrition' is widely recognised. Recently, the nutritional needs of hospital patients in particular have been the subject of close scrutiny. It is necessary to understand something of the basic nutrients in order to apply the principles of 'good nutrition' to everyday practice, whether in hospital or at home. The more important of these are briefly described below, together with common foods in which they occur. Further details of the functions of these and other nutrients are described on pp. 118 to 135.

Protein

This is essential for the manufacture and repair of many body tissues (e.g., muscles, hair, nails, etc.). It is also needed for the production of other vital body components such as enzymes, hormones and antibodies.

Protein is found in meat, poultry, fish, eggs and milk (including many milk products for example, cheese and yoghurt). Significant amounts of protein are additionally provided by nuts, pulses (haricot beans, lentils, etc.) and cereal containing foods including bread.

Carbohydrates

These provide energy and heat for the body and are necessary for the efficient metabolism of proteins and fats. Some carbohydrates also provide a valuable source of roughage as well as containing minerals and vitamins.

Carbohydrates can be subdivided into starches, fruits and vegetables and sugars:

1 Starches (bread, potatoes, rice, pasta, biscuits, breakfast cereals, etc.) are an important group of foods: in addition to giving heat and energy they also supply some protein, essential minerals and vitamins and roughage (especially if wholegrain varieties are used). They should not be omitted from the diet unless an extremely rigid reducing diet has been medically prescribed for a specific patient.

2 *Fruits and vegetables.* Ideally fruits (apples, pears, oranges, berries, etc.) should be included in the diet in their fresh form, not canned in syrup (see below). Fruits also provide Vitamin C and some roughage. Vegetables (carrots, beetroot, sweetcorn and other starchy varieties) can be fresh, frozen, canned or dried. Freezing vegetables does not affect the nutrient content significantly. Vitamin loss occurs readily during the cooking and preparation period however (see p. 6) and therefore great care should be exercised at this time.
NB Green leafy vegetables (e.g., cabbage and cauliflower, etc.) do not contain significant amounts of carbohydrate.

3 *Sugars* (sugar, glucose, jam, marmalade, all types of syrup, sweets, soft drinks, etc.) are not an essential part of the daily diet because, generally, they only contribute energy (or calories) but little else in the way of nutrients.

NB Milk also contains a significant amount of carbohydrate but, on account of its high protein content, it is generally classified as a protein containing food.

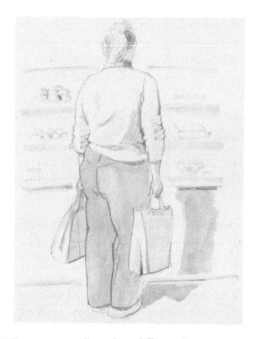

Fig. 2.1 Will one more really make a difference?

Fats

These are needed in order to protect the vital organs and maintain normal growth and development. They also provide fat soluble vitamins and essential fatty acids in addition to increasing the palatability of the diet. They are a highly concentrated source of energy (calories).

Fats are found mainly in butter, margarine, cream, egg yolks, cheese, fatty bacon and other fatty meats as well as in all types of oils. It should also be remembered that fats form an important part of many cooking processes.

Minerals

A large number of these are known to be essential to life and most of them are widely distributed in foods. The most important of these when considering dietary availability are calcium and iron.

1   *Calcium* is needed for the formation of healthy teeth and bones. It is also important in the blood clotting mechanism and the maintenance of neuromuscular stability.

Calcium is found in milk, hard cheese (e.g., Cheddar, Stilton, etc.), eggs and white bread. Significant amounts of calcium are present in the tap water in hard water areas (e.g., London).

2   *Iron* is a vital factor in the formation of haemoglobin. A deficiency of iron can cause anaemia.

Iron is present in red meat and offal (especially liver), eggs, bread, dried fruits and baked beans.

It is unlikely that dietary deficiency of any other minerals will occur because they are widely distributed in most commonly eaten foods. The functions of some of the other essential minerals and trace elements are discussed on pp. 132 to 135.

Vitamins

These are complex substances which, as their names implies, are vital for life. They can be divided into fat soluble vitamins and water soluble vitamins and each individual vitamin has one or more specific functions.

Fat soluble vitamins. These are found in fatty foods and are comparatively unaffected by various cooking and storage methods. They can be stored by the body and, in normal circumstances, deficiencies are unlikely. It should be noted that the

absorption of these substances is seriously reduced by the concurrent administration of mineral oils (e.g., liquid paraffin).

1   *Vitamin A* is essential for the maintenance of healthy epithelial
tissue and the prevention of night blindness. It is found in milk,
butter, margarine, egg yolk, hard cheese, liver and oily fish (e.g.,
herrings, sardines, etc.). The precursor of Vitamin A (carotene) is
found in green leafy vegetables and coloured vegetables and fruits
(e.g., carrots, tomatoes, apricots, etc.).

2   *Vitamin D* together with calcium is necessary for the development of healthy bones and teeth. Major dietary sources of Vitamin
D include eggs, margarine, fortified yoghurt, fortified evaporated
milk, oily fish and liver. It can also be synthesised from ultraviolet
light (sunlight) on the surface of the skin.

3   *Vitamins E and K* are widely distributed in foods and are only
required in comparatively small amounts by the body. It is
unlikely, therefore, that any problems will occur due to a dietary
deficiency.

Water soluble vitamins. These require careful consideration in
the average diet because the body does not retain large stores of
water soluble vitamins. It is also very important to realise that they
are much less stable than their fat soluble counterparts. Water
soluble vitamins are readily destroyed by prolonged exposure to
air, soaking and, finally, by cooking and during the serving
process.

1   *Vitamin B complex* is vital for the metabolism of carbohydrates.
Folic acid, Vitamin B_6 and Vitamin B_{12} are also necessary for the
formation of red blood corpuscles and deficiencies of any of these
substances can lead to anaemia. The chief dietary sources of this
group of vitamins are liver, yeast and green leafy vegetables.
Individual vitamins in the group are not otherwise supplied by the
same individual foods.

2   *Vitamin C* (also called ascorbic acid) contributes to the
efficiency of the immune system and is needed additionally for the
formation of various intercellular substances. It is widely distributed in all fruit and vegetables (particularly near the surface
under the skin). Potatoes, blackcurrant juice and citrus fruits (e.g.,
oranges, grapefruit, etc.) are particularly useful sources of this
vitamin.

Roughage

This is also known as dietary fibre and has recently been acknowledged to play an important role in the human diet. Roughage is formed from the indigestible matter found in plant structures and there are two main sources:

1 Cereals – particularly wholegrain. This includes bread and any other products made from flour (e.g., biscuits, breakfast cereals, pasta and rice).

2 Fruits, vegetables and nuts, including pulses, such as lentils and baked beans, which have a particularly high roughage content. Fruits and vegetables should be eaten in their skins whenever possible.

The function of roughage is to stimulate the lower gut to produce a soft, formed stool which is easy to pass. This is possible because the indigestible fibre swells in the gut and absorbs water thus adding bulk to the intestinal contents which then stimulates peristalsis.

Water

Water is an essential and often forgotten component of the diet. All the bodily processes take place within a fluid environment. It is, therefore, important that water (or similar clear fluids) should form a routine part of the daily dietary intake.

The average daily intake of fluid is approximately 2 litres and 1 litre of this will be derived from the fluid which occurs naturally in food.

NB It should be remembered that many ill patients will require at least 3 litres of fluid each day to compensate for fluid losses associated with specific disease states. If this level is not achieved and maintained, dehydration may follow with serious metabolic consequences.

Nutritional requirements of different groups of people

It is well established that different groups of people need different types and amounts of food. This is determined by various factors including sex, age and activity. Reference tables are available which provide guidelines to the levels of specific nutrients which are required during the life cycle (see Appendix III). These differences should be observed while individuals are in hospital and in most cases it is possible to adapt the main menu to incorporate any modifications which are necessary.

There are four criteria which should be particularly remembered when a hospital patient's requirements for nutrition are assessed:

1 Age
2 Activity and disease state
3 Ethnic background and/or moral convictions
4 Concurrent drug therapy

Age

There are times during the life cycle when more or less nutrition is needed. This should be considered in addition to any other dietary modifications which are requested for hospital patients.

Children. Childhood is a period of growth, particularly in infancy and during the early teens. There are increased requirements for protein, energy, minerals (particularly calcium) and vitamins (particularly Vitamin D).

If a child is very young, it may be necessary to modify the texture of the food (e.g., purees, soft foods, etc.) so that it can be managed more easily. The size of the portions and the types of food should be related to the particular age group — remembering that children can be rather conservative in their choice of foods.

Pregnancy. Obstetric patients have specific nutritional needs which must be met in order to protect foetal growth and development. There is an increased requirement for protein, energy, calcium, iron and vitamins and the relative increases vary according to the stage of the pregnancy (see Appendix III).

There may be occasions when it is advisable to alter mealtimes slightly or to modify the amount of food which is given at each meal. *There is no need to ensure that the expectant mother eats enough for two* before her baby is delivered.

Lactation. There is, again, an increased need for all the nutrients mentioned in connection with pregnancy. It is very important that meals should be served attractively to encourage the mother to eat at a time when she may not feel hungry.

Elderly. The nutritional requirements of the elderly, although slightly reduced, are extremely important. Elderly patients differ enormously from each other and should each be considered individually. In many cases physical handicap may govern their ability to eat. The following points should be remembered:

1   *Energy* – the total volume of food should provide enough energy. This may mean giving high energy supplements to those patients who are not able to eat large quantities of food.

2   *Texture* – many elderly people have impaired chewing ability and are unable to manage some foods.

3   *Fibre* – constipation and associated problems are a common cause for concern in the elderly. Make sure that there is enough fluid and fibre-rich food in the diet.

4   *Vitamins* – particularly Vitamin C and Vitamin D – are likely to be taken in insufficient amounts (see p. 6 for sources of these nutrients).

Activity

It is fairly obvious that the degree of physical activity of an individual will directly affect his dietary requirement for energy. It is important to remember that the level of activity may be quite different when he is a patient in hospital and that the dietary intake may need to be modified appropriately.

It is also important to remember that certain disease states can affect the need for various nutrients, especially protein and energy. Further information about this can be found on p. 15.

Ethnic background and/or moral convictions

NB These are not generally considered to be therapeutic diets and should be ordered through the hospital catering department. Most catering departments do not have the facilities to produce these special meals in the hospital kitchens, but a variety of suitable frozen meals can be obtained from commercial manufacturers.

Religious dietary constraints. Most hospitals have patients from a variety of ethnic backgrounds. Many religious sects believe that certain foods should not be eaten and these beliefs should always be respected while such a patient is in hospital.

HINDUS. Some Hindus are completely vegetarian (see p. 11) but most Hindus only avoid beef and beef products because the cow is believed to be a sacred animal. This includes items such as minced beef (beefburgers, etc.), corned beef, beef sausages and dishes cooked in beef dripping and in beef stock.

MUSLIMS. All Muslims avoid pig meat and all pork products as the pig is traditionally considered to be dirty. Some Orthodox Muslims will additionally only eat 'halal' meat (this term applies to the way in which the animal has been slaughtered). In many cases, however, Kosher meat is an acceptable alternative.

Both Hindus and Muslims are accustomed to eating significant amounts of starch in the form of rice or unleavened bread. They eat small amounts of meat and obtain much of their protein from pulses such as lentils and dried beans. There is a judicious inclusion of mild, aromatic spices in their diet and yoghurt is taken regularly.

ORTHODOX JEWS. All Jews avoid eating pig meat and all pork products including sausages, tinned meats, bacon and ham. Non-

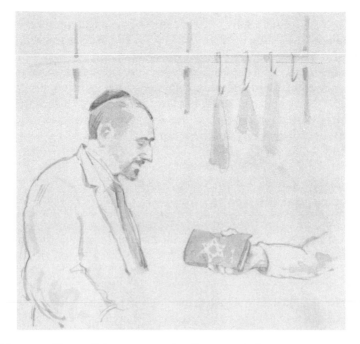

Fig. 2.2 Many religious sects practice dietary restrictions

orthodox Jews will eat the regular hospital diet if an alternative to these foods is provided.

Orthodox Jews, however, will not eat any meat which has not been slaughtered in a carefully prescribed manner (Kosher meat). The meal must, additionally, be prepared by an Orthodox Jew. Extremely strict rules govern their eating habits and it is essential to make sure that no one touches the patient's food apart from the patient himself. This also applies to the cutlery. If special Kosher meals are purchased by the hospital, the Catering Department will be able to advise further about the constraints governing their use.

It should also be remembered that Orthodox Jews will not take meat and milk at the same meal unless there is a guarantee that separate cooking utensils are always used. Therefore it would be inappropriate to offer a cup of milky tea with a Kosher meal.

Moral dietary constraints

Vegetarians. There are varying types of vegetarians and their dietary classifications are as follows:

NON-MEAT EATING. These patients will eat any meal providing it does not contain meat (this normally also includes poultry) or meat products such as lard, stock and gelatin.

It should be ensured that the patient's eating habits do have a genuine moral foundation — rather than a mere dislike of hospital meat!

LACTO-OVO-VEGETARIANS. These patients will not eat meat, poultry or fish or any products containing them. The protein in their diets is derived mainly from dairy sources and eggs.

LACTO-VEGETARIANS. This group will not eat meat, poultry, fish and eggs together with any products containing them. They will eat milk and milk products (including cheese, yoghurt and ice-cream).

Vegans. There is a minority of patients who refuse for either religious or, more usually, moral reasons, to eat any food which has an animal origin i.e., meat, poultry, fish, milk, cheese and eggs. The essential protein which they need is derived from pulses, nuts and cereals. Many Catering Departments are unable to provide complete vegan meals, but a suitable compromise can usually be reached after discussing the problem with the patient.

Vegetarian and vegan patients are generally well informed about food and the sources of various nutrients and it is comparatively unusual to see clinical signs of nutritional deficiencies in these groups. However, it is important to monitor their nutritional intake carefully. Protein, iron, calcium, Vitamin B_{12} and Vitamin D should be assessed with particular caution.

Concurrent drug therapy

The administration of drugs can also affect the nutritional status of a patient in addition to relieving the symptoms of a specific pathological condition. This can occur in several ways:

By altering the type and amount of food which is eaten:
1 Changes in the senses of smell and taste
2 Increased or decreased appetite
3 Drug administration can induce nausea and vomiting which will depress the appetite still further.

By altering the way in which nutrients are absorbed:
1 Modified gut motility
2 Changed secretion of digestive juices and enzymes
3 Damaged mucosal cells in the GI Tract
4 Formation of complex drug–nutrient substances which cannot be properly metabolised by the body.

By altering nutrient metabolism and excretion.

These points should be considered in the context of individual patients and it should also be remembered that most drugs have different effects on different people. Appropriate steps should be taken to rectify any possible nutritional deficiencies as early as possible in consultation with the medical and pharmaceutical staff. It is impossible to generalise about appropriate nutritional therapy in respect of most individual drugs, although guidelines for the use of MAOI drugs are detailed on p. 108. *If there is any doubt the doctor and/or pharmacist should always be consulted.*

How can the principles of good nutrition be applied in normal practice?

The theory and practice of any subject are very different and nutrition is no exception. It is not always practical to assess an individual's intake in respect of each nutrient and then decide whether or not this will be adequate.

The easiest way to overcome this problem is to use the concept of food groups and to ensure that *at least 2 helpings are taken from each group each day*:

Group 1	Group 2
Milk and dairy foods including	*Meat and fish, etc.* including
Milk (1/2 pint) Cheese Yoghurt	Meat Poultry Offal Fish Eggs Nuts Pulses (peas, dried beans, lentils)

Group 3	Group 4
Fruit and vegetables including	*Cereals* including
Citrus fruits (oranges, grapefruit) Apples Berry fruits Tomatoes Salad vegetables Potatoes Leafy vegetables (spinach, cabbage) Root vegetables (carrots, parsnips)	Bread (white, brown or wholemeal) Rice Breakfast cereals (preferably wholegrain) Pasta (spaghetti, macaroni) Biscuits

The use of food groups as outlined above can be applied with equal benefit to both the healthy and the sick. There are, however, many constraints which operate against people eating adequately while they are patients in hospital and these will be discussed in more detail in the next section.

Nutritional problems of patients in hospital

The problems of hospital starvation and/or iatrogenic malnutrition have been extensively reviewed recently in medical and
nursing literature. There is now no doubt that this phenomenon
not only exists but is alarmingly widespread in many hospitals. It is
important to recognise that the problem may be present at a local
level and to realise the implications of ignoring the need for an
adequate daily nutritional intake. This has been dealt with on a
more medically orientated basis in Chapter 6. There are, however,
certain practical considerations which must always be remembered
and which should be applied to each individual patient.

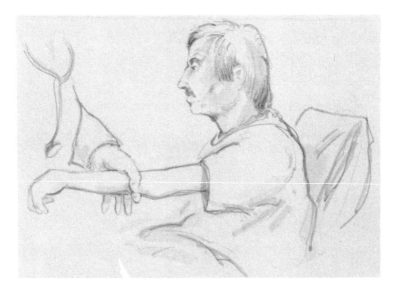

Fig. 2.3   Malnutrition i. common in hospital patients

No patient should be allowed to go without food in hospital unless
starvation has been prescribed specifically in connection with
particular surgical or medical procedures. Prolonged lack of
nutrition can give rise to clinical deficiencies of individual
nutrients. There are also more serious consequences which include
electrolyte imbalances, dehydration, loss of lean body mass,
increased susceptibility to infection and even death. It is, therefore,
of vital importance to everyone – not least the patient – to ensure
that he receives adequate nourishment *on a daily basis*. There are
three further points which must always be remembered:

1   The patient may have been malnourished before admission to hospital. This is particularly relevant when the diagnosis is one of a chronic disease state, for example, cardiac valve disease, carcinoma, intestinal failure, etc.

2   Individual requirements for specific nutrients and for energy may be *increased* in the presence of certain disease states such as burns, infections, etc.

3   Receiving food and actually eating it are two entirely different exercises. It is always necessary to check that the patient eats what he is offered!

Awareness of the possibility of nutritional depletion is vital to the subsequent management and well-being of the patient. This statement cannot be overemphasised. If attention is paid to the nutritional status of the patient at the earliest opportunity then he will demonstrate an improved response to treatment with an earlier discharge from hospital. *Any* doubts about any individual patient's diet should be referred to the medical staff immediately.

How do patients starve in hospital and what can be done to prevent it?

The immediate priority is to make sure that the patient is eating as well as can be reasonably expected. It is only when this has been ascertained that the need for any dietary manipulation (e.g., the provision of supplementary foods) can be assessed.

It is useful to remember the following points when making an initial estimate of a patient's eating ability and nutritional requirements:

1   **Who is responsible for making sure that the patient is adequately nourished?** In most cases this is the responsibility of the ward sister. The task of checking menu cards and supervising the patient at mealtimes, however, can often be delegated to a junior nurse who may not have enough nutritional knowledge to be able to make a reasonable assessment of the patient's dietary needs and relate them to his actual intake.

2   **Choosing from the menu.** Many hospitals now operate a system whereby the patient can select which items he wishes to eat. The patient should be encouraged to do this whenever possible; it will generate an interest in food and he will then be more

motivated to eat. Supervision and encouragement are essential at this stage.

3 **'Off Days'.** Everybody (including patients) has days when they do not feel like eating. If this is an isolated incident it should be no cause for serious concern but the situation should be monitored carefully.

If there is consistent difficulty in persuading a patient to eat adequately then the medical staff *must* be informed at once.

NB Experience has shown that the judicious use of alcohol – especially dry sherry – may stimulate the appetite. *Medical permission must be obtained first* and then alcohol can be brought in by relatives or written up on the drug chart if its use has been indicated.

4 **Between-meal snacks.** Many patients are given gifts of food by visitors. Try to ensure that these have some nutritional value such as fresh fruit, nuts, etc., rather than providing 'empty' calories e.g., sweets. It would be preferable to suggest that, for example, fresh fruit juice or a blackcurrant drink should be brought in, which contain some Vitamin C, rather than fizzy drinks which only contain calories.

A sick person's appetite is easily sated and it is important to remember that tea and biscuits could 'fill' a patient to the extent that meals may not be wanted. Soup also prevents hunger without necessarily providing adequate nutrition. Few nurses have ever been in hospital as patients and even fewer have experienced this within the year before commencing their training. It is, therefore, difficult to appreciate the problems which confront a patient. This is especially relevant when food is considered.

Most healthy people are apprehensive about any serious illness. A hospital patient is not only ill but has also been placed in a totally alien environment which can be frightening and sometimes even threatening. He is surrounded by doctors, nurses and other strangers who, occasionally, seem to speak a different language and who are, almost invariably, in too much of a hurry to explain the present situation clearly to him. He is subjected to strange tests and asked to take unfamiliar pills. Perhaps he may even be wearing strange bedclothes. It is easy to see how this situation can represent the total loss of an individual's security. The only factor with which he can expect to be familiar is the food. Unfortunately this is rarely the case!

There are many additional aspects which have to be remembered when considering why a particular patient is not eating well, some are patient-orientated and some are hospital-orientated. It is important to be able to differentiate between them in order to be able to manage each problem appropriately.

Anxiety. It is unusual for a hospital patient not to be extremely anxious and this has two basic causes:

1 *Worry about the reason for hospitalisation.* This is an obvious problem (see above) and a great deal of anxiety can be allayed by careful, sympathetic explanation. This is particularly important when a specific procedure has been proposed. It should be remembered that patients are often in a mild state of shock and are only capable of assimilating small items of information at a time. Information provided by a doctor on a ward round, for instance, is frequently misunderstood because it has been only partly heard.

2 *Worry about the home situation.* This may not even be mentioned by the patient. The fact that life has to continue at home while the patient is in hospital is something which is often overlooked.

Timing of meals. Most hospitals tend to serve the main meal in the middle of the day; many people normally eat their main meal in the evening. The meal itself may take a completely different form – particularly with the increased availability of fast foods and the consequent tendency to eat 'snacks'.

Unfamiliarity of the food. This may be manifest in several ways:

1 The description of a dish may not be understood (e.g., Carbonnade of Beef, Manchester Tart, etc.)

2 Unfamiliar cooking methods (e.g., use of different herbs and seasonings, etc.)

3 Unacceptable cooking methods (e.g., the patient may like rare roast beef, but would refuse to eat well-cooked roast beef).

In each case the patient may either not select a meal in the first place or not eat it when it arrives at mealtime.

Religious beliefs. It is well known that various religious sects will not eat particular foods (see p. 9). This should always be respected in the hospital situation and an appropriate alternative arrangement should be made. The Hospital Catering Manager should be involved whenever possible.

Dental state. Many people wear dentures. If complete dentures are worn, the patient will only retain approximately 35 % of his original chewing ability. This will have a significant effect upon the beginning of the digestive process. In practice many sets of dentures are kept in a mug on the bedside locker and are only worn for the ward round! The reason for this should be ascertained and it may be possible to organise a visit to the hospital dental department. It is also important to make sure that appropriate soft, nutritious food is available.

Anorexia. This could be due to several causes, all of which should be carefully considered:

1   Drug therapy – many drugs can precipitate loss of appetite as well as interfering with the absorption of specific nutrients (see also p. 12).

2   The patient may just be having an 'off day' (see p. 16).

3   There may be some underlying worry or fear that has not been identified by the hospital staff or even, perhaps, by the patient himself.

Instruction. Many people are not aware of the importance of food. The need for adequate nutrition is increased when an individual becomes ill and is admitted to hospital. This has to be emphasised to each patient.

It is of course necessary that the nursing staff are aware of the importance of nutrition. If a nurse is not convinced about this, she will not find it easy to convince a patient!

Organisation. Unfortunately, it is very unusual for mealtimes to be the only event taking place on a ward. Shift changes, drug rounds, ward rounds, staff breaks and other activities contribute to less emphasis being placed upon close supervision of the patient at mealtimes. Such supervision should include:

1   Confirmation that the patient has received the meal which was ordered.

2   Confirmation that the meal is attractively presented and served at the correct temperature.

3   A check to ensure that the meal is placed within physical reach of the patient and that appropriate cutlery, etc. has been provided.

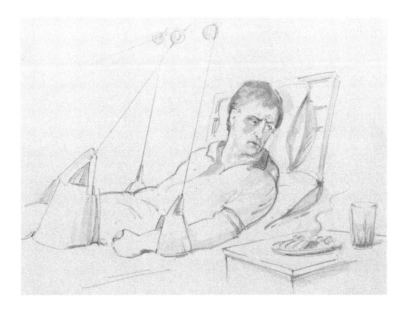

Fig. 2.4   Can the nurse help?

4   Help to feed the patient if he is unable to do this for himself. (The League of Friends or Voluntary Services Department may be able to help in this respect if there is a shortage of nursing staff.)

5   A check to ensure that the meal has been eaten and, if not, how much has been left. *This information should form part of the routine nursing report* and should be charted if necessary.

Medically prescribed procedures. Many tests involve starvation e.g., special X-rays, minor surgical procedures, etc. This should be remembered when the tests are ordered, particularly if the patient is undernourished. If a succession of such procedures is ordered and there is concern about the patient's nutritional status *then the medical staff must be advised immediately.*

It is easy to understand why patients may not feel like eating while they are in hospital. It is vital to make sure that every effort is made to overcome the problems which cause this. An awareness of the difficulties which exist is the key to their solution. Advice should be sought from all the personnel who are involved in the care of an individual patient whenever it is appropriate to do this. It may be necessary to request the help of professionals in other disciplines with the advantage that a concerted team approach to the problems of 'hospital starvation' will ensure that it does not occur and that each patient will receive the maximum benefit from his medical treatment.

What is a diet?

It is well recognised that the individual's need for various nutrients alters during the life cycle — a teenager will have different requirements from either an elderly person or a toddler (see Appendix III). Bearing this in mind a 'diet' can then be defined in the following terms:

A 'normal' diet is the daily intake of a range of foods which will provide enough of the essential nutrients to promote and subsequently maintain good health.

This is what anyone eats — whether he is well or sick. In the context of a hospital environment it is the food which is provided on the main menu to patients or in the staff canteen. It is usually prepared by the hospital Catering Department in the main hospital kitchens.

A 'modified' diet is the daily intake of a range of foods in which the intake of one or more of the essential nutrients has been modified. The purpose of a dietary modification is to ease the workload of a damaged or diseased organ (e.g., low protein diet in renal failure). A dietary modification is also used to control symptoms of a specific disorder (e.g., carbohydrate and/or energy modification in cases of diabetes mellitus).

A modified diet (or '*Special*' or '*Therapeutic*' diet) is specifically prescribed for an individual patient and a Dietitian will usually be involved. The food is generally prepared by specially trained cooks in a Diet Bay attached to the main hospital kitchens.

It is important to remember that not all hospitals have immediate access to specialist Dietetic facilities. Even if Dietitians are available it is still necessary for the nursing staff to have some knowledge of the various types of modified diets which are currently used. It is also extremely important that nurses should know about the principles of basic nutrition and the constraints which exist when feeding patients in hospital (see p. 13–20). The subsequent sections of this text will deal with various aspects of modified diets, providing adequate information for the nursing staff on the ward to be able to cope with some of the more usual dietetic problems which can arise on a day-to-day basis.

It must be stressed that if a Dietitian is available her advice should always be requested at the earliest opportunity. A Dietitian has specialist training and experience in tailoring the personal preferences of a patient to the specific constraints which are demanded by a therapeutic dietary modification.

Therapeutic diets

It is often difficult to ensure that a patient eats an adequate amount of food while he is in hospital (see p. 14). These difficulties may be compounded by modifying his diet in order to improve his medical condition and/or nutritional status. Diets can be modified in three ways:

1 The texture of the food can be altered
2 The nutritional content of the food can be adapted
3 The texture *and* the nutritional content of the food can be modified.

The first category of dietary modification may only be a short-term undertaking (e.g., post-operative feeding). Nevertheless it is important to make sure that the nutritional requirements of the patient are supplied appropriately. These types of modification are explained in further detail in pp. 24–36.

Long-term dietary manipulation is a continuing component of the patient's medical treatment. The need to observe various restrictions will continue after discharge from hospital and will then become part of the patient's lifestyle at home. This can present many difficulties in terms of food preparation and general way of life. It is vitally important that a dietitian is involved at the earliest stage possible. It is the dietitian who has the knowledge and specialist skills which are needed when any long-term dietary changes are proposed. She will be able to review the patient's regular eating habits (and those of his family) and advise how any changes can be effected. This includes detailed explanations of the reasons for a specific dietary prescription, the use of suitable food exchanges and discussion of appropriate cooking methods. She is also able to evaluate the success of any dietary manipulation by means of follow-up appointments with the patient and, if necessary, his family.

The following sections of this text are intended only as a guide. They provide possible solutions to some of the problems which may occur at ward level.

If there are any doubts regarding any patient and a dietitian is not available, the medical staff must be advised immediately.

There are some general points which should always be remembered when a patient has been prescribed a therapeutic diet:

1   A therapeutic diet is medically prescribable and any order for a diet must, therefore, be signed by a qualified member of the medical staff. If this practice is not followed there could be serious legal consequences.

2   A therapeutic diet constitutes an integral part of the medical or surgical management of the patient and his condition can be expected to improve as a result of the dietary prescription. It is, therefore, essential that all the required dietary modifications should be clearly understood and carefully observed.

3   The patient may have many questions about his diet; failure to answer these as soon as possible will lead to confusion and lack of co-operation (see also p. 17). If a question cannot be answered immediately, make sure that the patient knows that someone will come to see him shortly in order to explain his queries.

4   Therapeutic diets often involve daily restrictions of various foods (e.g., milk, butter, etc.). If this is the case these foods should be weighed out at the beginning of the day, labelled with the patient's name and the current date and kept separately from other routinely used foods.

5   Visitors often wish to bring in gifts of food for patients. They should be advised of the foods which are suitable and those which are unsuitable in respect of any patient receiving a therapeutic diet.

6   It is important to check the patient's bedside locker regularly to make sure that no unsuitable foods are either purchased from the League of Friends' trolleys, brought in by visitors or 'inherited' from other patients.

7   In some cases it may be necessary to record various aspects of a patient's dietary therapy. Remember to *weigh patients regularly,*

record fluid intake and output accurately and maintain any other appropriate charts as requested.

8   In most cases therapeutic diets are specially prepared for individual patients. If there is any alteration in the dietary prescription or if the patient is discharged *it is important to inform the appropriate staff immediately*. Apart from the food which could be wasted it may be necessary to arrange a follow-up appointment once the patient has been discharged.

9   A therapeutic diet should *only* be given to the patient for whom it has been specifically prescribed. It should *never* be used for anyone else.

3
Modified Diets I. Diets Modified in Texture or Consistency

There are several aspects to be considered when deciding how to feed a patient. General nutritional requirements may vary widely between individuals (see Appendix III). This may have nothing to do with their state of health. The type of food which is acceptable may also vary greatly (see p. 17). These limitations must be recognised when feeding patients in hospital because their nutritional status may already be compromised as a result of a pathological condition.

Some patients may be unable to eat 'normal' food despite the fact that there are no other restrictions placed upon their intake. Examples might include the very young and the very old. There are also many other categories of patient who may require some dietary modification in terms of the consistency or texture of their food. It must be remembered that there is not, necessarily, a need to modify the amounts of any of the nutrients which they require.

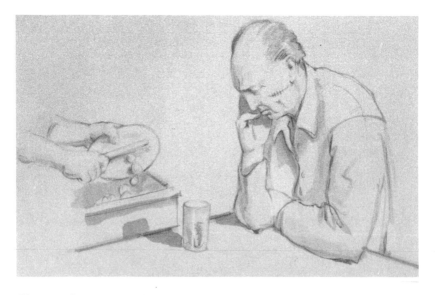

Fig. 3.1 Some patients don't want to eat . . .

The texture of food can be modified in the following ways:

1 Light (gastric/bland)
2 Soft
3 Purée
4 Full fluids
5 Clear fluids

Arrangements for implementing these modifications will, of course, vary from hospital to hospital. In many cases however, the majority of these categories can be managed by liaising with the Catering Department and advising them of the particular needs of individual patients.

Some hospitals have facilities which enable small quantities of food to be cooked at ward level. There can be little doubt that this is very helpful when dealing with individual patients. However, a central kitchen can also provide the appropriate foods. Take care to ensure that the appropriate staff are given as much advance warning as possible when any special modifications are required.

Light diets (including 'Bland' and 'Gastric')

It is unusual for a 'gastric' diet to be prescribed specifically. This form of treatment has been superceded by more effective drug therapy.

Aims

1 To enable a patient to maintain his nutritional intake despite various constraints

Physical or mental handicap
General debility
Poorly fitting dentures

2 To rest the gut when necessary e.g., post-operatively, during radiation therapy.

3 To avoid indigestion or the recurrence of other gastro-intestinal symptoms e.g., ulcer, 'Dumping' syndrome, etc.

Relevant drugs

These will vary according to the diagnosis of individual patients
but may include

1   Anti-emetics e.g., Chlorpromazine, Domperidone, Prochlor-
perazine, Promethazine Theoclate, etc.
2   Antacids e.g., Sodium Bicarbonate, compound proprietary
antacids
3   Antispasmodics e.g., Atropine Sulphate, Metoclopramide
hydrochloride
4   Ulcer healing drugs e.g., Carbonoxolone Sodium, Cimetidine

Important!

1   Meals should be served regularly with snacks in between. The
portion size will depend upon the patient's requirements but should
not be too large.

2   Meals should be neither too hot nor too cold and should be
attractively presented.

3   Fried foods and spiced or strong foods should be *avoided*.

4   Smoking and alcohol may aggravate gastrointestinal disturbances and should be discouraged.

5   The patient should be encouraged to eat slowly and chew his
food well. Drinking with meals should be *avoided*.

6   Many patients will know which foods can be tolerated and
which foods will aggravate any symptoms and should be avoided.

General

The following foods may cause problems and should be *avoided* if
there is any doubt about them:

1   Fried foods
2   Highly seasoned foods
3   Wholemeal breads, cereals and biscuits (it may be possible to
re-introduce these gradually at a later date)
4   Dried fruits and fruits with pips
5   Raw vegetables particularly cucumber
6   Onions
7   Cooked cheese

There is usually no need to sieve or purée foods.

Light diet: Menu modification

Breakfast	Cereal	Yes	Cornflakes, Porridge, Rice Krispies, etc.
	Fruit or fruit juice	No	
	Egg, bacon or fish	Yes	Not fried: white fish only
	Bread or roll & butter	Yes	White only*
	Marmalade or honey	Yes	'Jelly' type marmalade only Avoid 'comb' honey
	Tea or coffee and milk	Yes	Weak only
Mid-morning	Bread or roll & butter	Yes	White only*
	Jam or honey	Yes	Jelly type jam only. Avoid comb honey
	Plain biscuits	Yes	Rich Tea or Marie type only. Avoid wholegrain biscuits e.g., digestive
	Tea or coffee & milk	Yes	Weak only
Lunch	Soup	Yes	'Cream' types only
	Meat, fish,	Yes	Not fried or highly
	eggs or cheese		seasoned
	Potatoes or rice	Yes	Boiled or creamed only
and	Vegetables-all types	Yes	Watch onions, celery, sweetcorn, etc.
	Puddings	Yes	Watch those made with wholemeal flour
Supper			No dried fruit
			No skins or pips of fruit
	Tea or coffee & milk	Yes	Weak only
Mid-afternoon	Bread or roll & butter	Yes	White only*
	Jam or honey	Yes	See above
	Plain biscuits	Yes	See above
	Tea or coffee & milk	Yes	Weak only
Bedtime	Plain biscuits	Yes	See above
	Milky drink	Yes	
	Tea or coffee & milk	Yes	Weak only

* Some patients may be able to manage brown or wholemeal bread without any adverse effects.

Soft diets

This is similar to a light diet in many respects and the two categories are often confused. There is much greater uniformity of texture when a soft diet is used. The indications for a soft diet are sometimes similar to those for a light diet and the main differentiating factor is the physical state of the patient and the fact that he is able to tolerate more highly seasoned foods.

Aims

1   To enable a patient to maintain his nutritional intake despite various constraints

Physical or mental handicap
General debility
Poorly fitting dentures or no teeth
Partial obstruction of the oesophagus
Inflamed mouth

2   To rest the gut when necessary e.g., post-operatively, during radiation therapy, etc.

3   To avoid indigestion or the recurrence of other gastrointestinal symptoms.

Relevant drugs

These will vary according to the diagnosis and condition of individual patients. They may include

1   Anti-emetics e.g., Chlorpromazine, Domperidone, Prochlor-perazine, Promethazine Theoclate, etc.
2   Antacids e.g., Sodium Bicarbonate, compound proprietory antacids, etc.
3   Antispasmodics e.g., Atropine Sulphate, Metoclopramide hydrochloride, etc.
4   Ulcer healing drugs e.g., Carbenoxolone Sodium, Cimetidine
5   Analgesics
6   Antibiotics

Soft diets: Menu modification

Breakfast	Cereal	Yes	Porridge or similar cereal only
	Fruit juice	Yes	Watch acidity
	Fruit	Yes	*Soft* tinned or fresh fruit only
	Egg	Yes	Soft boiled, poached or scrambled
	Fish	Yes	White only
	Bacon, etc.	No	
	Bread or roll & butter	Yes	White only
	Marmalade or jam	Yes	'Jelly' type only
	Honey	Yes	Avoid 'comb' type
	Tea or coffee & milk	Yes	Weak only

Mid-morning	Bread or roll & butter	Yes	White only
	Jam or honey	Yes	See above
	Plain biscuits	Yes	Marie or Rich Tea type only; no wholegrain varieties e.g., digestive*
	Tea or coffee & milk	Yes	Weak only

Lunch	Soup	Yes	'Cream' types only
	Meat	Yes	Minced or *very* soft
	Fish	Yes	Baked in sauce or *very* soft, white only
and	Cheese	No	Unless in sauce
	Eggs	Yes	
Supper	Potatoes or rice	Yes	Boiled/creamed only
	Vegetables	Yes	Soft varieties only: no hard, woody stems, no skins or pips, no raw vegetables
	Puddings	Yes	No hard fruits or dried fruits. No skins or pips.
	Cheese & biscuits	No	
	Tea or coffee & milk	Yes	Weak only

Mid-afternoon	Bread & butter	Yes	White only
	Jam or honey	Yes	See above
	Plain biscuits	Yes	See above *
	Tea or coffee & milk	Yes	Weak only

Bedtime	Plain biscuits	Yes	See above*
	Milky drink	Yes	
	Tea or coffee & milk	Yes	Weak only

* Some patients may be able to manage plain biscuits – especially if they are encouraged to 'dunk' them in tea or coffee

Important!

1   Meals should be served regularly with snacks in between.

2   The texture should be uniformly soft, but not necessarily puréed; meals should be attractively served and should be neither too hot nor too cold.

3   Food should be carefully seasoned to ensure that each dish is recognisable but *very* 'hot' food seasonings should be avoided (e.g., ginger, chilli, etc.).

4   Nutritional intakes should be carefully monitored to ensure that deficiencies of energy, protein, iron and vitamins (particularly Vitamin C and Vitamin D) do not arise.

NB   It is normally necessary to add water to food in order to soften it; this 'dilutes' the nutritional content of the meal.

General

1   Many items on the main menu e.g., milk puddings, some soups and some main course dishes, will be suitable for patients requiring a soft diet.

2   Fruit juices and blackcurrant drinks are a useful source of Vitamin C.

3   Try to make sure that all the food and drinks which are offered to the patient are nutritious; avoid the inclusion of too many sugary snacks.

4   The patient may be aware of particular foods or flavours which he is unable to tolerate. These should be excluded from the diet.

Puréed diets

If a puréed diet is required all foods should approximate the consistency of baby food.

Aims

1 To enable the patient to maintain his nutritional intake despite difficulties in eating

No teeth e.g., after dental clearance
Severely inflamed mouth
Oesophageal obstruction
Extreme physical or mental handicap
General debility

2 To encourage the patient to eat while resting the gut e.g., post-operatively or during aggressive treatment e.g., radiotherapy.

3 Achievement of nutritional intake in infants.

Relevant drugs

These will vary greatly according to the specific diagnosis and condition of the individual patient. They may include

1 Anti-emetics e.g., Chlorpromazine, Domperidone, Prochlorperazine, Promethazine Theoclate, etc.
2 Antispasmodics e.g., Atropine Sulphate, Metoclopramide hydrochloride, etc.
3 Analgesics
4 Antibiotics
5 Chemotherapeutic agents

Important!

1 The intakes of energy, protein, Vitamin D, Vitamin B complex, Vitamin C and iron should be carefully monitored. Relevant supplementation should be medically prescribed if necessary and given as an elixir.

2 Patients receiving treatment for cancer are particularly likely to experience altered perceptions of taste (e.g., patients receiving chemotherapy often complain that milk tastes rancid). This should be recognised and catered for if at all possible.

3   The patient will probably feel fairly ill and will need to be encouraged to eat. Every effort should be made to ensure that the meal is attractively presented. Meals should be tasty but very 'hot' seasonings and spices should be avoided. The importance of a positive approach to the dietary limitations cannot be overstated.

4   High calorie/high protein supplements (especially drinks) should be encouraged.

5   Weigh the patient regularly.

6   Make sure that normal food (not puréed, etc.) is available as soon as the patient is ready to eat it.

7   If puréed food is being given to infants then the specially formulated baby foods should be used in preference. *All heavy seasoning and sweetening should be avoided.* The total requirement for nutrition will depend upon the age and size of the infant and should always be specifically calculated for each individual.

General

1   Tinned baby food may be included in the diet as an alternative to puréed meat and vegetables. It should not be used exclusively without appropriate nutritional supplementation.

2   Alcohol is a useful appetite stimulant and a small glass of dry sherry just before meals also provides a psychological 'boost'. *This must only be given after medical consent has been obtained.*

3   Milky drinks can usually be made up at ward level. It is advisable to try to vary the flavour and temperature as much as possible.

4   High calorie supplements which have no taste or sweetness should be used whenever possible. Further information about these should be available from

Department of Nutrition and Dietetics
Pharmacy
Catering Department

5   Make sure that dishes are seasoned enough to make them recognisable. Highly seasoned foods are not usually advisable.

Puréed diet: Menu modifications

Breakfast	Cereal	Yes	Thin or puréed porridge, Redybrek, etc. only
	Fruit or fruit juice	Yes	Fruit juice only; check that it is not too acidic
	Egg	Yes	Raw in milk or very lightly boiled or scrambled
	Bacon or fish	No	
	Bread or roll & butter	Yes	Only if the patient can manage it
	Marmalade or honey	Yes	'Jelly' type marmalade only Avoid comb honey
	Tea or coffee & milk	Yes	Weak only

Mid-morning	Milky drink	Yes	
	Plain biscuits	No	
	Bread & butter	Yes	If the patient can manage it
	Jam	Yes	'Jelly' type only
	Tea or coffee & milk	Yes	Weak only

Lunch	Soup	Yes	'Cream' type, strained only
	Fruit juice	Yes	If not too acidic
	Meat or fish	Yes	Puréed only with sauce or gravy
and	Eggs or cheese	Yes	*Lightly* cooked only
	Potatoes	Yes	Creamed only
	Vegetables	Yes	Puréed only
Supper	Puddings	Yes	Milk pudding, jelly, yoghurt, ice cream, puréed non-acidic fruits only
	Tea or coffee & milk	Yes	Weak only

Mid-afternoon	Milky drink	Yes	
	Plain biscuits	No	
and	Bread & butter	Yes	If the patient can manage it
	Jam		'Jelly' type only

Bedtime	Tea or coffee & milk	Yes	Weak only

Full fluids

This regimen supplies the patient with a complete and concentrated form of nutrition which is sufficiently liquid to pass down a straw.

Aims

1 To provide the patient with adequate nutrition while he is unable to eat any normal foods

Wired jaws
Oesophageal stricture
Following facial surgery
Acute oral or upper gastrointestinal inflammation
Following extensive major surgery

2 To prevent the need to pass a nasogastric tube or feed the patient parenterally.

Relevant drugs

These will vary according to the diagnosis and general condition of each individual patient.

Important!

1 The nutritional intakes of iron and Vitamin C should be monitored and supplemented if necessary.

2 A careful check should be kept on the patient's weight and general condition. A gradual return to normal foods should be encouraged as soon as possible.

3 Many patients may take a longer time than usual to drink their food. Allowances should be made for this.

4 Drug therapy may distort taste appreciation; this should be considered and catered for if appropriate.

5 Patients on these regimens often feel nauseated; they should be encouraged to take their food despite this and a positive approach to the problem is extremely important.

Full fluids: Menu modification

Depending on local arrangements these will either be sent up from the kitchen or will be prepared at ward level. The following points will always apply:

1 The fluid meal should be free from any lumps and should be liquid enough to pass down a straw.

2 It should be stirred thoroughly to remove any sediment before it is offered to the patient.

3 Careful attention should be paid to ensure that there is adequate variety of colour, flavours, temperature and taste.

4 If a 'meal' is rejected it should be discarded immediately to avoid any risk of bacterial contamination.

General

1 Supplements of high protein/high calorie fluid drinks should be given at ward level. These may be based on any of the following:

Milk and milk powders
Commercial products e.g., Complan, Build-Up, Fortimel, Ensure, Frutein, etc.
Soups
Fruit Juices
Eggs
Yoghurt
Ice Cream, etc.

Examples of some basic recipes are listed on Appendix V.

2 Alcohol is a useful appetite stimulant and a small glass of dry sherry just before meals also provides a psychological 'boost'. *This must only be given after medical consent has been obtained.*

Clear fluids

These are only given in specific circumstances and for a very short period e.g.

Pre-operatively
Post-operatively
As preparation for special diagnostic tests.

NB   The following fluids *only* should be given (*no other foods are allowed*)

1   Tea or coffee (no milk) — lemon and sugar are allowed
2   Fruit squashes
3   Mineral waters
4   Clear soups
5   Clear jellies

These regimens are nutritionally inadequate and should only be prescribed for the minimum period of time.

Important!

Elemental (no residue) formulae are suitable for inclusion in these regimens. Despite their nutritional completeness they are extremely unpalatable and are not recommended. For further information please refer to p. 110.

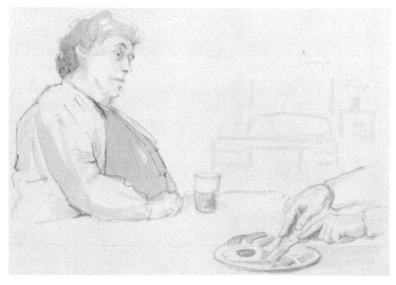

Fig. 3.2 Fluid diets can be nutritious (see p. 34)

4

Modified Diets II.
Diets Modified in Nutritional Content

In addition to considering the basic nutritional requirements of individual patients (p. 24) and, possibly, altering the consistency of the food which is presented, it may also be necessary to modify the content of the nutrients themselves.

Therapeutic diets such as those which follow *are prescribed in respect of individual patients*. Dietary prescriptions and meal plans should never be used for any patient other than that for whom it was specifically designed. There may, however, be occasions when it is necessary to implement a dietary prescription immediately and when a dietitian may not be available e.g., at weekends.

The following section is designed to be used *only* in the short term because it is impossible to be specific to individual patients in a text such as this. These are guidelines only and will certainly require modification for long-term use if the patient is to extract the maximum benefit from his dietary prescription and associated drug therapy.

It will be much easier to understand the next section of the text if the following points are noted.

Prescription. A therapeutic diet is medically prescribable and no patient should be given a diet without the necessary medical authorisation.

Relevant drugs. In most cases a selection of drugs which are commonly used in the treatment of a specific condition are mentioned. The lists are not intended to be exhaustive.

Meal patterns. These are based on the average type of meals and snacks which would be served in most hospitals.

Other information.

1 Important!
Some aspects of particular regimens are especially important and appear before the meal plan and modifications.

2 General
This covers the remaining details which are necessary to ensure the satisfactory management of a therapeutic diet in the short term.
    This text is not intended to replace individual diet sheets and is not, therefore, exhaustive in respect of any diet.

General. Each hospital has its own way of dealing with therapeutic diets and any local policies and procedures should always be considered *before* implementing any of the recommendations outlined subsequently.

Calorie Controlled Diets

Diabetic

Introduction

Diabetes Mellitus is a condition which is characterised by the inability of the body to utilise sugar. There are two types of Diabetes Mellitus:

1 **Insulin Dependent Diabetes (Type I).** This is also known as *juvenile onset diabetes* and is caused by the failure of the pancreas to secrete insulin. This is seen more commonly in young people and is treated by the administration of insulin (either by injection or in a continuous sub-cutaneous infusion).

2 **Non-insulin Dependent Diabetes (Type II).** This is also called *maturity onset diabetes* and occurs in older people. The pancreas produces insulin but in insufficient quantities. Diabetic symptoms are usually controlled by diet alone or by diet together with oral hypoglycaemic tablets and/or especially formulated guar gum preparations.

The diet is a vital part of the management of any diabetic patient and dietary limitations must always be observed closely.

Dietary fibre and the diabetic diet

Diabetic diets have been traditionally restricted in total carbohydrate or energy (calories) or both. There has also been a requirement for insulin depending upon the type of diabetes (see p. 38). Recent developments in medical research indicate that this is not the most effective way to control the blood sugar levels of a diabetic.

Carbohydrates occur in two main forms:

1 Simple sugars (e.g., sugar, sweets, etc.)
2 Complex starches (e.g., bread, potatoes, etc.)

Starches are broken down into simple sugars during the digestive process after which they are absorbed into the blood stream. This takes longer than the straightforward absorption of those foods which are already in the form of simple sugars.

If large quantities of simple *sugars* are eaten they will enter the bloodstream fairly quickly and cause the blood sugar level to rise rapidly. This will require more insulin in the short term to enable absorption into the cells to take place, thereby restoring the blood sugar level to the normal range.

The breakdown products of *starches* on the other hand will take longer to enter the bloodstream, the blood sugar will rise less quickly and less insulin will be needed.

It has also been shown that the fibrous nature of the complex carbohydrates slows down the absorption rate and the consequent need for insulin still further. Whenever possible, therefore, high fibre containing forms of these carbohydrates should be included in the diet.

The dietary management of the diabetic is undertaken with this principle in mind and places much greater emphasis on a comparatively large intake of the complex carbohydrates with an associated raised intake of dietary fibre.

Aim

To reduce the blood sugar to a normal level and to maintain a constant blood sugar level thereafter. This is effected by:

1 Modifying the carbohydrate intake – complex carbohydrates are digested more slowly than simple sugars and help to maintain blood sugar levels within an acceptable range.

2 Restricting the energy intake if necessary – many diabetics with non-insulin dependent diabetes are overweight. Reducing the body weight helps to control the symptoms of diabetes.

Relevant drugs

1   Short acting soluble insulins (usually 2 or 3 injections daily) e.g., Actrapid, Velosulin, Neusulin.
2   Intermediate acting insulins (usually 2 injections daily) e.g., Rapitard, Semitard, Insulatard.
3   Intermediate acting insulins with short acting insulin (usually 2 injections daily) e.g., Initard, Mixtard.
4   Long acting insulins (1 injection daily) e.g., Lente, Monotard, Lentard, Neulente.
5   Continuous insulin infusion

Short term – in acutely ill diabetics – usually administered by intravenous infusion via a Sage pump. Short acting soluble insulin is given and is titrated against blood sugar levels.

Long term – in well controlled diabetics – administered by a subcutaneous infusion pump. The regimens vary according to the requirements of individual diabetics.

6   Oral hypoglycaemic drugs. These fall into two groups and are given in tablet form:

Sulphonylureas e.g., Tolbutamide, Chlorpropamide, Glibenclamide
Biguanides e.g., Metformin, Phenformin

NB   A diabetic may not always require drug therapy but should *always* have a dietary prescription.

Important!

1   Carbohydrate (CHO). This includes all sugary and starchy foods (see p. 39) and also milk and fruit.

2   Distribution of CHO and energy (calories). These *must* be spaced evenly through the day.
    It is particularly important to give the correct amount of CHO at each meal to a diabetic receiving insulin.
    If the diabetic refuses to eat what has been sent up, the CHO allowance should be made up to the prescribed amount using the portions on p. 48.

3   If a diabetic is being treated with soluble insulin it is important to ensure that he receives a meal approximately 30–45 minutes after his injection for optimal blood sugar control.

4   Diabetics should never be sent for tests e.g., X-rays, if it is likely that their meals may be delayed or even missed completely as a

result. This will probably cause them to have a hypoglycaemic reaction (hypo). This is particularly important if a diabetic is receiving insulin.

5 The following charts represent a basic guide *to be used in the short term only*. It is essential that a diabetic should be seen by a dietitian in order that his diet can be correctly calculated.

6 An adequate intake of dietary fibre should be encouraged for better diabetic control (see below). For further information about fibre containing foods see p. 56.

7 Make sure that details of the diabetic's dietary distribution are clearly displayed – preferably at the end of the bed.

8 No sugar is allowed.

Guidelines for visitors

It is very important that visitors should be fully aware of any dietary limitations which have been prescribed. They should be encouraged to bring in non-edible gifts e.g., flowers, books, writing paper, etc. This may not always be possible in which case the following items could be suggested:

Diabetic and low calorie fruit squashes. **NB** No other diabetic products are allowed if the total energy (calories) has been restricted

Slim-line and other low calorie mineral waters

Soda water

Bovril, Oxo, Marmite or bouillon cubes (to make hot drinks at ward level)

Tomato juice, Pure Lemon Juice (PLJ)

Salad vegetables e.g., tomatoes, cucumber, etc.

Blackberries, blackcurrants, bilberries, grapefruit, gooseberries, lemons, melon, rhubarb (any cooked fruit should be stewed without sugar – use a sweetener if necessary)

Artificial sweeteners e.g., Sweetex, Saxin, Canderel, Hermesetas in tablet or liquid form

Diabetic: Menu modifications

These guidelines should be used together with the relevant distribution charts which appear on the following pages:

Breakfast	Cereal	Yes	*See chart* – preferably whole-grain e.g., Shredded Wheat or Weetabix. *No* sugar. Use milk from daily allowance
	Fruit or fruit juice	Yes	*See chart.* Tomato juice allowed freely
	Egg or cooked breakfast	Yes	*No* fried foods if calories are restricted.
	Bread or roll	Yes	*See chart.* Preferably wholemeal
	Marmalade, honey	No	Diabetic marmalade only allowed if no calorie restriction
	Butter or margarine	Yes	
	Tea or coffee	Yes	With milk from daily allowance
Mid-morning	Bread & butter	Yes	*See chart* – preferably wholemeal
	Jam or honey	No	See above
	Plain biscuits	Yes	*See chart* – preferably wholemeal e.g., digestive
	Tea or coffee	Yes	With milk from daily allowance
Lunch	Clear soup	Yes	*See chart* for other variations
	Meat, fish, cheese or eggs	Yes	Average portions but no pastries or sauces
	Potatoes, rice, pasta	Yes	*See chart* – *Not* fried or roasted if calories are restricted
and	Green leafy & salad vegetables	Yes	
	Root and pulse vegetables	Yes	
Supper	Puddings	Yes	See chart: 1 portion equals a) Fresh fruit *or* b) Cheese and 2 biscuits *or* c) Small (5oz) carton natural yoghurt *or* d) 2 ice cream brickettes
Mid afternoon	Bread and butter	Yes	*See chart* – preferably wholemeal
	Jam or honey	Yes	Diabetic jam only allowed if *no* calorie restriction

	Plain biscuits	Yes	*See chart* — preferably whole-meal e.g., digestive
	Tea or coffee	Yes	With milk from daily allowance
Bedtime	Bread and butter	Yes	*See chart* — preferably wholemeal
	Jam or honey	No	See above
	Plain biscuits	Yes	*See chart* — preferably whole-meal e.g., digestive
	Milky drink	Yes	*See chart* — use milk from daily allowance
	Tea or coffee	Yes	With milk from daily allowance
Daily	Milk	Yes	*See chart* — for use in tea, coffee, on breakfast cereal, etc.

General

1 In-between meal snacks should *not* be given unless they are specifically indicated on the diabetic's meal plan.

2 Diabetic or low calorie fruit squashes (specifically labelled 'suitable for Diabetics') and mineral waters only are allowed. All other soft drinks are *forbidden.*.

3 Artificial sweeteners in liquid or tablet form (e.g., saccharin, Saxin, Hermesetas) should be used instead of sugar in beverages. These may be obtained from the Pharmacy.

4 Diabetic jams, marmalades and other diabetic products may *only* be used if the patient is not overweight.

NB These products can have a laxative effect if they are eaten in excessive amounts.

5 *Make sure* that the patient does not have a supply of unsuitable foods hidden in his bedside locker and that visitors are aware of any dietary restrictions (see Guidelines for visitors, p. 41).

6 *Alcohol* is allowed in moderation if medical approval is obtained first. The patient should not drink on an empty stomach and the energy (calorie) value of the alcohol consumed should be included in the daily allowance.

NB Alcohol is not allowed if the total energy in the diet is restricted in order to encourage weight loss.

7 *Saturated fats* — the intake of this type of fat (see p. 72) should be restricted if *practical* and replaced with polyunsaturated fats.

Table 4.1 Diabetic meal plan: Distribution A. These meal plans should be used only for diabetics who are receiving: short acting insulins; intermediate acting insulins; insulin infusions; oral hypoglycaemic drugs; no drug treatment.

gCHO	Breakfast				Mid a.m.		Lunch				Mid p.m.		Supper					Bedtime		Daily
	Fruit or Cereal f. juice	Egg	Bread roll(s) or Plain biscuits	Bread (slices)	Plain biscuits	Bread (slices)	Meat, fish, eggs, or cheese	Potato (scoop of creamed)	Bread (slices)	Pudding	Plain biscuits	Bread (slices)	Thickened soup	Meat, fish, eggs, or cheese	Potato (scoop of creamed)	Bread (slices)	Pudding	Plain biscuits	Bread (slices)	Milk
100	NO	NO	YES	1	1	NO	YES	1	NO	1	2	NO	NO	YES	1	NO	1	2	NO	10 fl.ozs (300 ml)
120	YES	NO	YES	1	1	NO	YES	1	NO	2	2	NO	NO	YES	1	NO	1	2	NO	10 fl.ozs (300 ml)
140	YES	NO	YES	1	1	NO	YES	2	NO	2	2	NO	NO	YES	1	NO	2	2	NO	10 fl.ozs (300 ml)
160	YES	YES	YES	1	1	NO	YES	2	NO	2	2	NO	NO	YES	2	NO	2	2	NO	10 fl.ozs (300 ml)
180	YES	YES	YES	1	2	NO	YES	2	1	1	2	NO	NO	YES	2	NO	2	2	NO	10 fl.ozs (300 ml)
200	YES	NO	YES	2	2	NO	YES	3	NO	2	2	NO	NO	YES	2	NO	2	3	NO	10 fl.ozs (300 ml)

220	YES	NO	YES	2	NO	1	YES	3	NO	2	NO	1	NO	YES	3	NO	2	NO	1	YES	3	NO	2	3	NO	10 fl.ozs (300 ml)
240	YES	NO	YES	2	NO	1	YES	2	1	2	NO	1	NO	YES	3	1	2	NO	1	YES	2	1	1	3	NO	10 fl.ozs (300 ml)
260	YES	NO	YES	2	2	1	YES	2	1	2	YES	1	YES	YES	2	1	2	YES	1	YES	2	1	1	NO 1	10 fl.ozs (300 ml)
280	YES	NO	YES	2	2	1	YES	2	1	2	YES	1	YES	YES	2	1	2	YES	1	YES	2	1	1	1	10 fl.ozs (300 ml)

*** Are you looking at the right chart?? – check the drugs ***

Points to note:

1 These are arbitrary distributions and will need to be modified in respect of individual patients: please consult the dietitian

2 1 small scoop creamed potato = 1 potato (size of egg)   3. Condiments allowed freely (Unless specifically contra-indicated)

No sugar to be added under any circumstances

Table 4.2 Diabetic meal plan: Distribution B. These meal plans should be used only for diabetics who are receiving: long acting insulins.

gCHO	Breakfast				Mid a.m.	Lunch				Mid p.m.		Supper					Bedtime		Daily
	Fruit or f. juice	Cereal	Egg roll(s)	Bread (slices) or Plain biscuits (slices)	Bread (slices) or Plain biscuits (slices)	Meat, fish, eggs, or cheese	Potato (scoop creamed)	Bread (slices)	Pudding biscuits (slices)	Plain biscuits	Bread	Thickened soup	Meat, fish, eggs, or cheese creamed	Potato (scoop of creamed)	Bread (slices)	Pudding biscuits (slices)	Plain biscuits	Bread	Milk
120	NO	NO	YES	1	2	YES	1	NO	1	1	NO	NO	YES	1	NO	1	4	NO	10 fl.ozs (300 ml)
140	YES	NO	YES	1	2	YES	1	NO	2	1	NO	NO	YES	1	NO	2	4	NO	10 fl.ozs (300 ml)
160	YES	NO	YES	1	2	YES	2	NO	2	1	NO	NO	YES	2	NO	2	4	NO	10 fl.ozs (300 ml)
180	YES	NO	YES	1	2	YES	2	NO	2	NO	1	YES	YES	2	NO	2	NO	1	10 fl.ozs (300 ml)

200	YES	YES	YES	1	YES	2	NO	2	NO	1	YES	YES	2	NO	2	NO	4	NO	10 fl.ozs (300 ml)
220	YES	NO	YES	2	YES	2	NO	2	NO	1	YES	YES	2	NO	2	NO	2	1	10 fl.ozs (300 ml)
240	YES	NO	YES	2	YES	3	NO	2	NO	3	NO	YES	YES	2	1	2	3	1	10 fl.ozs (300 ml)

** Are you looking at the right chart? – check the drugs**

Points to note:

1 The bedtime snack must *never* be forgotten—otherwise the patient may go 'hypo' during the night

2 Condiments are allowed freely (unless specifically contra-indicated)

3 1 small scoop creamed potato = 1 potato (size of egg)

No sugar to be added under any circumstances

Carbohydrate exchanges

Every diabetic diet should be carefully calculated to ensure that a balance is maintained between dietary intake, exercise and available insulin. *It is vital that the prescribed amount of carbohydrate should always be taken if this has been indicated on the diet sheet.* Energy (calories) should be evenly distributed throughout the day otherwise.

If, for some reason, you have to make up the correct total of carbohydrate (e.g., too little is sent up from the kitchen, the diabetic refuses some food, etc.) the following portions may be helpful.

Each of the following foods contains 10 g carbohydrate

2/3 oz bread (brown or white)	1/2 roll *or* 1/2 slice from large loaf *or* 1 slice from small loaf
1/2 oz cereal	3 tablespoons *or* small bowl porridge
1/2 oz biscuits	2 plain e.g., Rich Tea, Marie, etc. *or* 1 Digestive
2 oz boiled or mashed potato	1 small scoop *or* 1 potato the size of an egg
2 oz cooked rice	1 tablespoon
1/3 pt milk	1 glass, whole *or* skimmed
5 oz natural yoghurt	1 small carton
2 oz vanilla ice-cream	2 small 'hospital' brickettes
2/3 oz unflavoured Complan	4 heaped teaspoons
1/2 oz Horlicks, Bournvita, Ovaltine or drinking chocolate	2 heaped teaspoons
4 oz unsweetened orange juice	1 small glass
4 oz eating apple	1 medium sized apple
5 oz orange	1 medium, weighed with peel
3 oz banana	1 small *or* 1/2 large, weighed with skin
5 oz Heinz cream of tomato soup	2/3 cup *or* 10 tablespoons
7 oz Heinz cream of chicken soup	a small tin holds 10 oz
8 oz Heinz cream of mushroom soup	a small tin holds 10 oz

Reducing

Introduction

Energy (or calories) is derived from four sources: proteins, fats, carbohydrates and alcohol. Energy is produced at the following approximate rates:

1 gram protein	= 4 kilocalories
1 gram carbohydrate	= 4 kilocalories
1 gram fat	= 9 kilocalories
1 gram alcohol	= 7 kilocalories

The amount of energy required by the body (and yielded by the various nutrients) is measured in kilocalories (kcals) but is generally referred to as Calories. An alternative unit, the kilojoule, is also used in some hospitals:

1 kilocalorie	= 4.2 kilojoules

To maintain constant body weight the energy intake should balance the energy expenditure. If this balance is upset then weight is either gained or lost as a result. Although many patients can manage on a reduced overall energy intake this must be carefully regulated to ensure that basic nutritional requirements are met (see p. 3–9). This generally means restricted intakes of fat, refined carbohydrate and alcohol.

The energy intake should be restricted only after considering the patient's usual consumption, energy expenditure and the desired weight loss. Low calorie diets should not be prescribed arbitrarily because individual requirements for energy vary so greatly (see p. 7). 'Crash' diets should be avoided whenever possible – consistent, slower weight loss is usually the more successful form of treatment. As a guideline the average person should lose weight satisfactorily on a daily energy intake of 1200–1500 Calories derived from a variety of foods.

Aims

1 To achieve weight loss by reducing calorie intake

2 To lower blood sugar levels when necessary e.g., non-insulin dependent diabetes, obesity.

Relevant drugs

1 Amphetamine-like drugs e.g., Fenfluramine, Diethylpropion and Mazindol are generally *discouraged*. Patients should be encouraged to understand the underlying cause of their obesity and to use their will-power.

2 Oral hypoglycaemic drugs e.g., Tolbutamide, Chlorpropamide and Phenformin may be prescribed for some mild diabetics.

Important!

1 Make sure that the patient (and his visitors) know what foods are allowed (see p. 51). Check the bedside locker regularly.

2 Remember to weigh the patient regularly.

3 Make sure that the daily allowances e.g., milk, bread, biscuits, etc. are carefully measured and labelled. *No extra items are allowed.*

4 Try and encourage the patient to eat three meals each day and to take as much exercise as is practical.

5 Maintain a positive, encouraging attitude towards the patient!

6 No sugar is allowed.

Guidelines for visitors

It is very important that visitors should be fully aware of any dietary limitations which have been prescribed. They should be encouraged to bring in non-edible gifts e.g., flowers, books, writing paper, etc. This may not always be possible in which case the following items could be suggested:

Diabetic and low calorie fruit squashes. **NB** No other diabetic products are allowed

Slim-line and other low calorie mineral waters

Soda water

Bovril, Oxo, Marmite or bouillon cubes (to make hot drinks at ward level)

Tomato juice. Pure Lemon Juice (PLJ)

Salad vegetables e.g., tomatoes, cucumber, etc.

Blackberries, blackcurrants, bilberries, grapefruit, gooseberries, lemons, melon, rhubarb (any cooked fruit should be stewed without sugar — use a sweetener if necessary)

Artificial sweeteners e.g., Sweetex, Saxin, Canderel, Hermesetas in tablet or liquid form.

General

1 *Only three portions of fruit are allowed each day.* This includes puddings at lunch and supper.

2 If the patient requires an artificial sweetener e.g., saccharin, Saxin, Hermesetas, etc., it may be possible to obtain this from the Pharmacy.

3 All diabetic products are forbidden with the exception of diabetic and low calorie fruit squashes and mineral waters.

4 Alcohol is *not* allowed in any form.

5 Some medicines e.g., cough syrups, contain large amounts of sugar and should not be used if they can be avoided.

6 The following foods are also *forbidden*:

Sugar and products containing sugar or glucose including:
    All puddings
    Sweets and chocolates
    Marmalades, jams and honey
    All sweetened fruit drinks including concentrates and squashes
    All sweetened mineral waters including Lucozade and Coca-Cola

Fats and all products containing significant amounts of fat including
    Fried foods
    Mayonnaise and salad cream
    Nuts (all types) and crisps
    Pastries and cakes

Thickened or other high calorie liquids including
    Thickened soups
    Complan, Build-up, etc.
    Ovaltine, Horlicks and other milky drinks

Reducing: Menu modifications

These guidelines should be used in conjunction with the distribution chart on p. 53.

Breakfast	Cereal		See chart
	Fruit or fruit juice	Yes	Unsweetened grapefruit and tomato juice allowed freely – otherwise from daily allowance.
	Egg or cooked breakfast		See chart – no fried or very fatty food allowed
	Bread or roll		See chart – preferably
		Yes	wholemeal
	Butter or margarine		See chart
	Marmalade or honey	No	
	Tea or coffee	Yes	Milk from daily allowance
Mid morning	Bread & butter	No	
	Plain biscuits		See chart
	Tea or coffee	Yes	Milk from daily allowance
Lunch	Clear soup	Yes	
	Meat, fish, cheese or eggs	Yes	See chart – no pastries, fried foods or sauces
and	Potatoes, rice, pasta		See chart – not fried
	Green leafy and salad vegetables	Yes	
	Pulse and root vegetables		See chart
Supper	Puddings	No	See chart 1 piece fresh fruit *or* 1 ice cream brickette *or* 1 small (5 oz) carton natural yoghurt
Mid afternoon	Bread & butter	No	
	Plain biscuits	Yes	See chart
	Tea or coffee	Yes	Milk from daily allowance
Bedtime	Bread & butter	No	
	Plain biscuits	Yes	See chart
	Milky drink	No	See chart – plain milk may be allowed
	Tea or coffee	Yes	Milk from daily allowance
Daily	Milk ⎫		See chart
	Bread ⎬	Yes	**NB** 3 plain biscuits may be exchanged for 1 slice bread (remember butter is restricted!)
	Butter ⎭		

Table 4.3 Reducing diet – distribution

Relevant drugs: Oral hypoglycaemic agents e.g. chlorpropamide, phenformin (Mild Diabetics only)

Calories	Breakfast			Mid a.m.	Lunch and supper					Mid p.m.	Bedtime	Daily	Daily
	Cereal	Egg	Bread-slices or Roll*	Plain Biscuits*	Meat or Fish or Cheese or Eggs	Green Leafy Veg.	Root Veg.	Potato (Plain Boiled)	Fresh Fruit	Plain Biscuits*	Plain Biscuits*	Milk	Butter
500	No	No	¼	No	Small	Large	No	No	1	No	No	3½ fl. ozs (100 ml)	¼ oz (8 gm)
800	No	Yes	1	No	Average	Yes	Small	No	1	1	1	7 fl. ozs (200 ml)	½ oz (15 gm)
1000	No	Yes	1	No	Average	Yes	Small	No	1	2	2	10 fl. ozs (300 ml)	½ oz (15 gm)
1200	Yes (no sugar)	Yes	1	2	Average	Yes	Small	1 Small	1	2	2	10 fl. ozs (300 ml)	½ oz (15 gm)
1500	Yes (no sugar)	Yes	1½	2	Average	Yes	Small	2 Small	1	2	2	15 fl. ozs (400 ml)	¾ oz (22 gm)

* Preferably wholemeal varieties

Points to note
1 Meat or fish or eggs but *no* pastry or sauce
2 Cheese at one meal only, preferably cottage cheese
3 See p. 51 for 'forbidden foods'
4 Do not give cheese and biscuits instead of a pudding
NB *No sugar or fried food is allowed under any circumstances*

Disorders of the Gastrointestinal Tract

Roughage and residue

There is considerable confusion regarding the nomenclature of these categories of diet. The following explanation may be helpful for the purposes of this text:

The total faecal content or residue has three main 'solid' constituents:

1 *Roughage* – this is the indigestible fibrous material found mainly in wholegrain cereal and plant foodstuffs. It passes through the intestine essentially unchanged.
2 *Intestinal secretions* – including various 'breakdown' products (e.g., red blood cells). Any food which increases these (such as fats) will add to the total faecal contents by various mechanisms which include slowing the transit time.
3 *Bacteria* – any diet which will minimise the substrate for bacterial proliferation will also reduce the faecal residue (e.g., milk is a substrate for bacterial proliferation and, therefore, a low residue diet should not contain any milk).

Modifications of roughage and residue

1 *High roughage* (also called *high fibre*).

Many gut ailments are caused by lack of stimulation of the gut wall. This, in turn, results from a small faecal bulk which is often difficult to pass. Associated conditions include constipation, haemorrhoids, varicose veins and diverticular disease.

A high roughage diet is considered to be generally beneficial for health and is advocated because of its protective effect against such chronic disease states as cancer, diabetes and coronary heart disease.

2 *Low roughage* (also called *low fibre*)

This is the most commonly prescribed diet for a variety of conditions when the mobility of the gut needs to be reduced e.g.

Preparation for barium enema
Preparation for EMI scanner tests
Mild intestinal inflammations

Roughage is composed of fibre from two sources which have to be excluded from the diet:

a   Cereal foods
b   Fruits, vegetables and nuts

Certain conditions may require that the fruit, vegetable and nut fibre components only are removed from the diet.

3   *Low residue*

This is not commonly used in the long term because it tends to be difficult to prepare and unpalatable to eat. It should not, therefore, be prescribed unless it is really necessary e.g.,

Preparation for bowel surgery
Acute intestinal inflammation

The dietary restrictions are the same as those for a low roughage diet with an additional modification: milk and all milk containing products are eliminated from the diet in order to reduce the faecal bulk to a minimum.

4   *No residue* (also called '*elemental*')

Technically it is impossible to achieve no residue because the faeces contain residual products of metabolism (e.g., degraded blood cells, etc.). It is, however, possible to eliminate all dietary residue by giving an 'elemental' diet. This is a formula preparation and further information is given on p. 110. The feeds must be used with great care and should be given under careful supervision. There are several indications for their use including:

As an alternative to intravenous nutrition

To rest the lower intestine – all the nutrition is absorbed in the upper half of the small intestine. This would be useful in cases of:

Bowel fistulae
Short bowel syndrome
Ulcerative colitis
Cröhns disease

Pre-operative preparation when it is important that the gut should be as clear as possible, but when the patient requires continuous complete nutrition.

What are the dietary sources of roughage (fibre) and how does it work in the body?

Recent medical research indicates that there are many advantages associated with a high fibre diet. It has been shown that several common pathological conditions e.g., varicose veins, haemorrhoids, diverticular disease, are associated with an inadequate fibre intake and that these illnesses can be avoided by simple dietary modification.

How much is 'enough'?

This will, obviously, vary between individuals but it is generally considered that most people could usefully increase the fibre content of their diet by approximately 50 %. This is especially true if the present dietary pattern indicates that no unrefined cereals are being included.

It is important to remember that bowel frequency is not only particular to each patient but that it is also affected by factors other than diet, such as stress or the amount of exercise which is taken.

Roughage or dietary fibre is derived from two major sources:

1 *Wholegrain cereals and any foods containing them* e.g.,

Wholemeal bread, rolls, crispbreads, etc.
Wholemeal biscuits e.g., digestives
Baked goods made with wholemeal flour e.g., cakes, pastries, puddings, etc.
Wholemeal pasta e.g., lasagne, macaroni, etc.
Wholegrain or 'brown' rice

These foods contain the 'whole' grain of the cereal as their name implies and this includes the outer husk or 'bran'. (Refined cereals do not include the outer husk — it is removed during the milling process.) It has been shown that this outer part of the grain is a source of many nutrients as well as providing the roughage which is needed by the gut in order for it to work properly.

2 *Fruits, vegetables and nuts including pulse vegetables* (e.g., peas, dried beans and lentils). The fibrous structure of these foods is not completely broken down by the human digestive system and, again, provides essential roughage.

NB Bran itself is widely available and may also be used to increase the fibre content of the diet (see p. 58).

The role of dietary fibre or roughage is to increase the intestinal bulk. This in turn stimulates peristalsis and the efficient elimination of the faecal contents.

The structure of fibre is such that it can absorb large quantities of water thus enabling an expansion of its original volume. (This concept can be more clearly illustrated by considering how grains of rice 'swell' and absorb water during the cooking process.)

It is, therefore, important to ensure that an adequate intake of fluid is achieved when a high fibre diet is prescribed. For further information see p. 58.

Bran

There may be occasions when an increased fibre (roughage) intake has been prescribed but when it is either impossible or impractical to persuade the patient to include enough high fibre foods in his diet. This approach should always be attempted initially because it is more beneficial for health in the long term.

Bran is the fibrous outer covering of each wheat grain. This is removed from the wheat grain during milling in order to produce white flour. Wholemeal flour is produced by retaining the bran with the wheat grain during the milling process.

Bran is commercially available in the form of small, light flakes which are either coarsely or finely ground. The coarse flakes are more beneficial than the fine flakes.

It is usually possible to obtain bran from either

Department of Nutrition and Dietetics
Catering Department
Pharmacy

If it is not available within the hospital it is stocked by most retail chemists, health food shops and many supermarkets.

How much bran should be given?

Initially 1 teaspoonful of bran should be taken with each main meal. This amount may need to be increased. This can be effected by adding 2 extra teaspoonfuls of bran daily until relief from constipation is obtained.

No more than 2 tablespoonsful of bran should be taken in one day without informing the medical staff.

How to use bran

In cooking – it can be included when making pastries, scones, cakes and bread, etc. It is not required if wholemeal flour is used.

As an addition to dishes:

Sprinkled over and stirred into breakfast cereals and puddings
Added to soups and stews
Stirred into milk, yoghurt or fruit juice

NB   Bran has a fairly strong flavour and the latter option above should be used with caution!

Bran should never be given to a patient by the spoonful!

Important!

1   *Fluid* – see p. 60. If bran is included in the diet it is very important that the patient should drink at least 2–3 pints (1–1½ litres) of fluid each day in the form of tea, coffee, water, minerals, fruit juices, squashes or soups.

2   *Remember* to warn the patient that he may experience some flatulence and abdominal discomfort initially, but that this should soon pass!

High roughage (high fibre)

This is not, normally, classified as a therapeutic diet and the main kitchen menu should be modified appropriately. If supplies of bran are required they should be obtained from

Department of Nutrition and Dietetics
Catering Department
Pharmacy (see p. 57 for further information.)

Roughage (fibre) is the indigestible fibrous component of two groups of foods:

1   Wholegrain cereals (including flour and products made with flour, wholegrain breakfast cereals, wholegrain pasta, brown rice)
2   Fruits, vegetables (including pulses e.g., peas, dried beans and lentils) and nuts.

High roughage (high fibre): Menu modifications

Breakfast	Cereal	Yes	Wholegrain only e.g., Shredded Wheat, All Bran, muesli
	Fruit juice or fruit	Yes	Preferably fruit
	Bacon, egg, fish, etc.	Yes	
	Bread or roll & butter	Yes	Preferably wholemeal
	Marmalade	Yes	Avoid 'jelly' types
	Tea or coffee and milk	Yes	

| **Mid morning** | Plain biscuits | Yes | Wholemeal e.g., digestive, oatmeal, etc. |
| | Tea or coffee & milk | Yes | |

Lunch	Soup	Yes	Preferably made from pulses/vegetables
	Meat, fish, cheese, eggs	Yes	
	Potatoes	Yes	In skins if possible
and	Vegetables	Yes	All types
	Pudding	Yes	Using wholemeal flour, etc. if possible
	Fresh fruit	Yes	
Supper	Tea or coffee & milk	Yes	

Mid afternoon	Bread & butter	Yes	Preferably wholemeal
	Jam	Yes	Avoid 'jelly' types
	Plain biscuits	Yes	Preferably wholemeal
	Tea or coffee & milk	Yes	

Bedtime	Plain biscuits	Yes	Preferably wholemeal
	Milky drink	Yes	
	Tea or coffee & milk	Yes	

| **Daily** | Milk | Yes | Allowed freely |
| | Butter | Yes | Allowed freely |

Aims

1 To produce well formed soft stools which are easy to pass.

2 To stimulate the gut into adequate peristaltic action to reduce/eliminate diverticulae.

Relevant drugs

None — laxatives should *not* be used in addition to a high fibre diet unless there is a *specific* indication for them.

Important!

1 Try to modify the fibre content of the diet before resorting to the addition of bran.

It is important to encourage patients to make long-term modifications to their eating habits to ensure a healthier lifestyle.

2 Fibre exerts an effect by absorbing water from the gut thereby increasing the faecal volume. *Make sure* that the patient drinks at least 2−3 pints (1-1½ litres) fluid each day in the form of tea, coffee, water, minerals, fruit juices, squashes or soups.

3 *Remember* to warn the patient that he may experience flatulence and some abdominal discomfort initially, but that this should soon pass!

4 Increase the fibre content of the diet *gradually*.

General

1 Porridge is not a good source of fibre unless extra bran has been added before serving.

2 This type of meal plan may also be followed by patients who have not been specifically advised to increase their intake of roughage.

Remember to check that there are no contra-indications.

3 It should not be necessary to use bran as well as a high roughage diet.

Low roughage (low fibre)

It is often possible to manage this dietary modification using the main kitchen menu. Roughage (fibre) is the indigestible fibrous component of two groups of foods:

1 Wholegrain cereals (including flour and products made with flour, wholegrain cereals, wholegrain pasta, brown rice, etc.)

2 Fruits, vegetables (including pulses e.g., peas, dried beans and lentils) and nuts.

Aim

To reduce the mobility of the gut by reducing the faecal bulk:

For diagnostic purposes using X-ray procedures e.g., barium enema.

To reduce mild intestinal inflammation.

To avoid strain post-operatively by reducing the frequency of defaecation e.g., rectal surgery, gender reassignment.

Relevant drugs

These will vary according to the patient's medical/surgical condition.

Important!

1 If the diet has been prescribed on a short-term basis for diagnostic purposes, it is prudent to order it for slightly longer than it is actually required.

2 Vitamin supplementation may be required if the diet has been prescribed for a longer period of time. It is advisable to check the intake of Vitamin C.

3 Some patients may know which foods upset them. If they are not specifically included on the guidelines on p. 62 they should be omitted anyway.

4 Sieving or puréeing vegetables does not remove the fibre!

Low roughage: Menu modifications

Breakfast	Cereal	Yes	No wholegrain cereals; Cornflakes, Rice Krispies, etc. are allowed
	Fruit (any type)	No	
	Fruit juice	Yes	If strained
	Egg, bacon, fish	Yes	Not fried
	Bread or roll	Yes	White only
	Butter and honey	Yes	
	Marmalade	Yes	'Jelly' type only
	Tea or coffee & milk	Yes	
Mid morning	Plain biscuits	Yes	No wholemeal – allow Rich Tea, Marie type, etc. only
	Tea or coffee & milk	Yes	
Lunch	Soup	Yes	Strained or clear varieties only
	Meat, fish, cheese or eggs	Yes	Avoid fried and highly seasoned dishes. Meat should be lean
and	Potatoes	Yes	Boiled or creamed only
	Pasta or rice	Yes	Not wholegrain or brown
	Vegetables (all types)	No	
	Puddings	Yes	Avoid those containing (a) Wholemeal flour, etc. (b) Fruit of any type
	Cheese and biscuits	Yes	No Vita Wheat, Ryvita, etc.
Supper	Tea or coffee & milk	Yes	
Mid afternoon	Bread & butter	Yes	White only
	Jam	Yes	'Jelly' type only
	Plain biscuits	Yes	Marie, Rich Tea type only
	Tea or coffee & milk	Yes	
Bedtime	Plain biscuits	Yes	No wholemeal – see above
	Milky drink	Yes	
	Tea or coffee & milk	Yes	
Daily	Milk	Yes	Allowed freely
	Butter or margarine	Yes	Allowed freely

General

1   Fried foods and highly seasoned foods: these do not necessarily contain roughage. However they tend to be rather indigestible and they can contribute to faecal formation (see below). It is advisable to *omit* them for these reasons.

2   Alcohol should only be taken with medical consent.

3   The *small* amounts of vegetables which are served in stews, etc. should do no harm provided that all other vegetables and fruits are omitted.

4   Certain regimens may require that only foods containing fruits, vegetables (including pulses) and nuts are eliminated from the diet. *In that case* only wholegrain cereals and foods containing them *would* be allowed in addition to those foods listed on the meal plan.

Low residue

This is not commonly used in the long term because it tends to be difficult to prepare as well as being unpalatable to eat. The following groups of foods all contribute to the total faecal residue and should, therefore, be *omitted*:

1   Wholegrain cereals (including flour and products made with flour, wholegrain breakfast cereals, wholegrain pasta, brown rice, etc.)

2   Fruits, vegetables (including pulses e.g., peas, dried beans, lentils, etc.) and nuts

3   Milk and all products containing milk (e.g. cheese, yoghurt, ice-cream, etc.) and any products made from milk (e.g., milk puddings) except for daily allowance, see p. 65

Aim

To clear the bowel of most of the faecal contents:

For diagnostic purposes e.g., colonoscopy, sigmoidoscopy, etc.
To reduce an acute intestinal inflammation e.g., ulcerative colitis, Cröhns disease.
To rest the gut e.g., after major colonic surgery.

Low residue: Menu modifications

Breakfast	Cereal	Yes	Cornflakes, Rice Krispies Milk from daily allowance
	Fruit (all types)	No	
	Fruit juice	Yes	Strained varieties only from daily allowance
	Egg, bacon or fish	Yes	Not fried
	White bread or roll	Yes	Use Marmite or honey as a spread
	Butter or margarine	Yes	From daily allowance
	Tea or coffee	Yes	With milk from daily allowance
Mid morning	White bread	Yes	Permitted spread only
	Butter or margarine	Yes	From daily allowance
	Plain biscuits	No	
	Tea or coffee	Yes	With milk from daily allowance
Lunch	Soup	Yes	Clear varieties only
	Lean meat, fish or egg	Yes	Cooked in permitted way only
	Cheese	No	Unless used as milk exchange
and	Potatoes	Yes	Boiled or mashed only
	Pasta or rice	Yes	Permitted varieties only – boiled only
	Vegetables (all types)	No	
Supper	Pudding	No	Unless (a) Plain jelly (b) Small milk pudding made with milk from allowance
Mid afternoon	White bread	Yes	Permitted spread only
	Butter or margarine	Yes	From daily allowance
	Plain biscuits	No	
	Tea or coffee	Yes	Milk from daily allowance
Bedtime	White bread	Yes	Permitted spread only
	Butter or margarine	Yes	From daily allowance
	Plain biscuits	No	
	Milky drink	No	Plain milk only is allowed if taken from daily allowance
	Tea or coffee	Yes	Milk from daily allowance

Daily Allowances	Milk (any type)	Yes	½ pint (300 ml) *only or* 1 oz (25 g) hard cheese e.g., Cheddar
	Butter or margarine	Yes	¾ oz (20 g) only
	Fruit juice	Yes	¼ pint (150 ml) *only* – strained only

Relevant drugs

These will vary according to the patient's medical/surgical condition. Vitamin supplementation may be required.

Important!

1 If the diet has been prescribed on a short term basis for diagnostic purposes it is prudent to order it for slightly longer than it is actually required.

2 Vitamin supplementation should be prescribed if the diet is required for more than a few days. *The intakes of both water soluble and fat soluble vitamins will be below the recommended levels.*

3 Remember to advise the patient that his faecal output will be considerably reduced.

4 Very few foods are allowed freely – see list below.

5 Make sure that the daily allowances of milk, butter, etc. are clearly labelled and carefully supervised.

General

1 All fried and highly seasoned foods should be *avoided.*

2 Remember to check the labels on any packets or tins of food e.g., Complan, Build-Up (which are not allowed!).

3 Alcohol should be avoided.

Low residue foods allowed freely

1 Lean meat, white fish, eggs (stewed, grilled, baked, poached, steamed or boiled only)

2 Potatoes (mashed or boiled only)

3 Spaghetti, macaroni, rice – *no* wholemeal varieties and boiled only

4 Bread and rolls (white only)
5 Breakfast cereals (refined only e.g., Cornflakes, Rice Krispies, etc.)
6 Drinks – Marmite, Oxo, Bovril
  Clear soups
  Soda water and other minerals
  Fruit squashes
  Fruit juices (strained only)
  Tea and coffee in moderation only
7 Plain jelly
8 Thin gravy, tomato purée
9 Honey, golden syrup, white sugar, artificial sweeteners
10 Boiled sweets, mints, marshmallows, Turkish Delight (nothing chocolate covered) only

---

'No' residue

The only successful way of reducing the bowel contents to a minimum while continuing to feed a patient orally is by giving an Elemental Diet. This type of diet is a formula preparation and further details regarding its administration can be found on p. 110. It is worth remembering that these diets are very expensive and unpalatable and should not be used as supplements.

Low fat

Fat is one of the essential nutrients and, as well as being a highly concentrated source of calories, also supplies fat soluble vitamins and essential fatty acids in the diet. It is usually possible (and advisable) to reduce the overall intake of dietary fat in the healthy individual without adversely affecting either the palatability or the nutrient content of the diet.

Aims

1   To reduce stimulation of an inflamed gall bladder e.g., cholecystitis, obstructive jaundice.

2   To prevent excretion of excessive amounts of fat e.g., steatorrhea.

Relevant drugs

There may be a requirement for fat soluble vitamins.

Important!

1   A 'low fat' diet will contain approximately 40 g fat. Although this can be reduced further *if really necessary*, a 'no fat' diet is not practical.

2   If the diet is prescribed as a short-term measure for diagnostic purposes, it is prudent to order it for slightly longer than it is actually required.

3   Vitamin supplementation will not be necessary in the short-term. If the diet is to be implemented on a long-term basis then the possible need for fat soluble vitamins should be considered.

4   Make sure that the daily allowances of milk, butter, etc. are clearly labelled and carefully supervised.

5   Energy requirements should be met by increasing the amount of carbohydrate in the diet. This should be derived from high fibre containing foods.

6   The following foods must be *avoided*:

Fried foods
Whole milk and products made with or from whole milk – use skimmed milk or skimmed milk powder instead. 'Filled' milk powders are *not* suitable substitutes – check the labels.
Butter or margarine other than the daily allowance (see p. 68).
Egg yolks – see allowances (p. 68).
For further fat containing foods please refer to the list on p. 69.

General

1   A low fat diet is often a case of personal preference without necessarily being prescribed medically. In these cases it is usually

Low fat: Menu modifications

Breakfast	Cereal	Yes	Use skimmed milk
	Fruit or fruit juice	Yes	
	Egg	No	
	Grilled bacon or white fish	Yes	Lean only – *No* oily fish e.g., kipper
	Bread or roll	Yes	White or brown
	Butter or margarine	Yes	From daily allowance
	Marmalade or honey	Yes	
	Tea or coffee	Yes	Use skimmed milk
Mid-morning	Bread	Yes	
	Butter or margarine	Yes	From daily allowance
	Plain biscuits	No	
	Tea or coffee	Yes	Use skimmed milk
Lunch	Soup	Yes	Clear soup or vegetable soup only – *no* cream soups
	Meat *or*	Yes	Lean only – grilled, boiled, stewed or roast (use inside slices *only*). *No* pastry
and	Fish *or*	Yes	White only – *no* sauce
	Cheese *or*	Yes	Cottage cheese *only*
	Egg	Yes	See 'Allowances'
	Potatoes or rice	Yes	Boiled only –no butter
	Vegetables or salad	Yes	All types
Supper	Pudding	Yes	Low fat yoghurt, jelly, fruit (any type) or skimmed milk puddings only
Mid-afternoon	Bread	Yes	White or brown
	Butter or margarine	Yes	From daily allowance (see mid-morning)
	Plain biscuits	Yes	2 only (any type)
	Tea or coffee	Yes	Use skimmed milk
Bedtime	Plain biscuits	No	
	Milky drink	No	Plain skimmed milk only is allowed
	Tea or coffee	Yes	Use skimmed milk
Daily	Milk	Yes	1 pint skimmed or 2 oz (50 g) skimmed milk powder
	Butter or margarine	Yes	1 oz (25 g) low fat spread may be substituted for ½ oz (15 g) butter
Weekly	Eggs	Yes	3 egg yolks only; egg whites are allowed freely

possible for the patient to select meals directly from the main menu.

2 Some patients may not be able to tolerate highly seasoned foods or strong tea and coffee. These foods should be omitted if it is appropriate to do so.

3 In addition to the items listed on p. 67 the following foods must also be *avoided*:

'Made-up' meat dishes e.g., pâté, liver sausage, hamburgers, sausages, etc.

Baked goods e.g., cakes, pastries or extra biscuits

Salad creams and dressings; lemon juice or vinegar may be used instead

Chocolates, toffees, marzipan or fudge. Boiled sweets, marshmallows, mints and Turkish Delight (no chocolate) are allowed.

Ovaltine, Horlicks and other similar beverages

Cream of any type

Nuts and crisps of any type

High protein

Protein is an essential nutrient without which the human body cannot survive for a prolonged period (see p. 3). The intake of protein can, however, be modified in the treatment of specific disease states (see p. 78).

Aims

1 To replace losses caused by protein–losing enteropathies.

2 To prevent tissue breakdown e.g., bedsores, fistulae, etc.

3 To restore nitrogen balance (and prevent negative nitrogen balance) in catabolic patients e.g., burns, post-operative, etc.

4 To replace the urinary excretion of protein e.g., nephrotic syndrome.

5 To compensate for dialysate losses of protein e.g., CAPD.

Relevant drugs

These will vary according to the individual disease state.

Important!

1   Any protein given to a patient must be utilised as effectively as possible and should not be used to provide energy (see p. 81). Energy needs, therefore, should be met from non-protein sources i.e. fat and carbohydrate.

A high protein diet should also be a high energy (high calorie) diet.

2   Many patients requiring a high protein intake have poor appetites and do not feel like eating large quantities.

Alternative methods of feeding should be used if appropriate.

Sip feeding − see p. 34
Tube feeding − see p. 141

3   Gentle persuasion is normally far more effective than any other means of attempting to encourage a patient to eat!

General

1   Encourage protein-rich snacks between meals whenever possible. Reduce the amount of food eaten at the main meals if this will help.

2   'Push' the meat or fish portion and potatoes at mealtimes rather than the vegetables. Similarly encourage cheese rather than biscuits if the patient feels unable to eat both.

3   Vary the type of protein offered as much as possible e.g., sandwiches, milk shakes, fortified soups, etc.

4   Most soups do not contain a lot of protein (although these may be what the patient prefers). Try to ensure that soups are fortified with milk powder, etc. whenever possible (see recipes in Appendix V). Bovril, Oxo and Marmite are not good sources of either protein or calories and only reduce the patient's ability to eat.

5   *Small* quantities of alcohol especially dry sherry may serve as an appetite stimulant. *This should only be given with medical consent.*

6   If the patient is mobile encourage him to take as much exercise as practical.

High protein (high energy): Menu modifications

Breakfast	Cereal	Yes	
	Fruit juice or fruit	Yes	Only if wanted
	Egg, bacon, fish, etc.	Yes	Double helping *if* practical
	Bread or roll	Yes	Double helping *if* practical
	Butter and marmalade	Yes	
Mid-morning	Bread & butter	Yes	As sandwich if possible
	Egg, cheese or meat	Yes	
	Milky drink	Yes	
Lunch	Soup	Yes	Encourage only if fortified or made from lentils, peas, etc.
	Meat, fish, eggs, cheese	Yes	Double helping if possible and practical
and	Potatoes	Yes	
	Vegetables	Yes	
	Pudding	Yes	Milk puddings, custard, ice cream and yoghurt are preferable
Supper	Cheese and biscuits	Yes	
Mid-afternoon	Bread & butter	Yes	As sandwich if possible
	Egg, cheese or meat	Yes	
	Milky drink	Yes	
Bedtime	Plain biscuits	Yes	
	Milky drink	Yes	
Daily	Milk	Yes	At least 1 pint (600 ml)

7 Drug round:

Casilan – if tolerated this could be given as a medicine (25 g daily in water or milk). It is very unpalatable and should only be used as a last resort (see Appendix V for other suitable products).

Hycal – this is a concentrated source of calories only. It is more palatable if it is served chilled (see Appendix V for other suitable products).

Prescribable high protein products – various preparations are available which are specifically indicated in conjunction with high protein diets. Further information should be available from

Department of Nutrition and Dietetics
Pharmacy

High energy/high calorie

Energy (or calories) are derived from proteins, fats and carbohydrates — see p. 3. High energy diets are, therefore, often high protein diets as well unless there is a medical indication to the contrary. Information about high protein diets can be found on p. 69.

The energy content of the diet can be increased in the following ways:

1 *Starches* — include more bread and cereal foods during the day. If the protein intake is to remain constant allow

$$1 \text{ oz meat} = 3 \text{ slices ordinary bread}$$

2 *Fats* — e.g., butter, oil, dripping, cream can be increased by:
Frying, sautéeing, roasting food
Adding butter to vegetables and on bread
Adding cream to soups, stews and puddings

3 *Sugars* — e.g., sugar, honey, jam, boiled sweets, etc. can be increased by
Adding to puddings, etc.
Eating suitable between-meal snacks

4 *High energy foods* — e.g., cheese, milk, nuts, etc. can also be encouraged as between meal snacks, although it must be remembered that they also contain significant amounts of protein.

5 *Pharmaceutical supplements* — several products are available which can be used in conjunction with this type of diet (see Appendix V). A particularly useful example is a glucose polymer which is readily soluble in water and has no sweetness (e.g. Polycal, Maxijul, Caloreen). Further information will be available from:

Department of Nutrition and Dietetics
Pharmacy

Gluten free

Gluten is one of the proteins which is present in wheatflour. Intolerance to gluten is characterised by skin disorders (e.g., dermatitis herpetiformis) and intestinal abnormalities (e.g., coeliac disease). The illness should be diagnosed positively before a gluten free diet is initiated.

Aim

To eliminate gluten from the diet thereby removing the acute allergic response which it causes.

Relevant drugs

Fat soluble vitamins and iron may be prescribed initially.

Important!

1   *All* products containing *wheatflour* must be eliminated from the diet. This includes bread, biscuits, pies, pastries and certain breakfast cereals.

2   A gluten free diet is usually a lifelong form of treatment. The patient should be fully aware of the importance of adhering to his diet − and any consequences which will arise if he cheats.

3   Remember to ensure that visitors are aware of the dietary limitations so that they do not bring in unsuitable gifts of food.

4   The patient may also be advised to avoid any products which contain rye, oats and/or barley.

5   Newly diagnosed patients tend to be poorly nourished. This should be corrected at the earliest opportunity.

General

1   Supplies of proprietary products which are gluten free should be available from

Department of Nutrition and Dietetics
Catering Department
Pharmacy
(This includes breads, biscuits and pasta.)

Gluten free: Menu modifications

Breakfast	Cereal	Yes	Cornflakes or Rice Krispies
	Fruit or fruit juice	Yes	
	Egg, bacon, fish	Yes	No breadcrumbs, etc.
	Bread or roll	No	Use gluten free bread *only*
	Butter & marmalade	Yes	
	Tea or coffee & milk	Yes	
Mid-	Bread or roll	No	Use gluten free bread only
morning	Butter and jam	Yes	
	Plain biscuits	No	Use gluten free biscuits only
	Tea or coffee & milk	Yes	
Lunch	Soup	Yes	Completely clear soups only are allowed
	Meat, fish, eggs or cheese	Yes	No gravies or sauces No made-up dishes No breadcrumbs
and	Potatoes and rice	Yes	Avoid croquette potatoes
	Pasta	No	Use gluten free pasta only
	Vegetables (all types)	Yes	
	Puddings	No	Milk puddings and ice cream (not macaroni or semolina) are allowed
Supper	Fruit (all types)	Yes	Custard is allowed
	Cheese and biscuits	No	Use gluten free biscuits (cheese *is* allowed)
	Tea or coffee & milk	Yes	
Mid-	Bread or roll	No	Use gluten free bread only
afternoon	Butter and jam	Yes	
	Plain biscuits	No	Use gluten free biscuits only
	Tea or coffee & milk	Yes	
Bedtime	Plain biscuits	No	Use gluten free biscuits only
	Milky drink	Yes	Bournvita or Complan only
	Tea or coffee & milk	Yes	

2   Check the patient's locker regularly to ensure that no unsuitable foods are being eaten.

3   Many commercial products are gluten free and carry a sign to indicate this. The sign represents a grain of wheat with a line crossing through it – indicating that wheat (and, therefore, gluten) is not present in the particular product.

Milk free

Intolerance to milk and milk products is usually apparent either as an acute gastrointestinal disturbance or as a more generalised reaction affecting the skin and breathing mechanisms. It is seen more commonly in children although transient milk intolerance sometimes occurs following surgery.

Aim

To eliminate milk and most milk products from the diet thus relieving any allergic response.

Important!

1 Patients may vary in their degree of intolerance; some may be able to eat products containing small amounts of milk e.g., biscuits, while others may need to eliminate milk completely.

2 There may be an intolerance of either casein (milk protein) or lactose (milk sugar) or both. If there is any doubt omit everything containing milk.

3 Many commercial products contain milk (particularly lactose) – these should be avoided. Check any labels carefully.

4 The following products should be completely eliminated from the diet:

Milk (all types including milk powders)
Cheese (all types)
Yoghurt
Ice cream
Cream

NB Butter is usually allowed – it contains only trace amounts of lactose. Margarine may not be allowed.

5 Many tablets contain lactose as a filling agent. Check that the patient is receiving lactose free medication.

6 Make sure that the patient and his visitors are fully aware of the implications of any dietary limitations – and the consequences of failing to observe them.

Milk free: Menu modifications

Breakfast	Cereal	Yes	No Special K
	Fruit or fruit juice	Yes	
	Egg, bacon, fish, etc.	Yes	No sausage
	Bread or roll	Yes	White or brown if known to be milk free
	Butter and marmalade or honey	Yes	No margarine
	Tea or coffee	Yes	
	Milk	No	Use substitute
Mid-morning	Bread or roll	Yes	See above
	Butter and jam	Yes	No margarine
	Plain biscuits	Yes	If known to be milk free
	Tea or coffee	Yes	
	Milk	No	Use substitute
Lunch	Clear soup	Yes	No cream soup
	Meat, fish, eggs	Yes	No milk or cheese based sauces
	Cheese	No	
	Potatoes or rice	Yes	No instant potato, no creamed or mashed potato
and	Vegetables	Yes	All types
	Pudding	Yes	No milk puddings, custard, ice cream, etc. Pastries and sponges must be made without milk
Supper	Fruit	Yes	All types
	Cheese and biscuits	No	
Mid-afternoon	Bread	Yes	White or brown if known to be milk free
	Butter and jam	Yes	
	Plain biscuits	Yes	If known to be milk free
	Tea or coffee	Yes	
	Milk	No	Use substitute
Bedtime	Plain biscuits	Yes	If known to be milk free
	Milky drink	No	
	Tea or coffee	Yes	
	Milk	No	Use substitute
Daily	Milk	No	Use a non-dairy creamer or alternatively Wysoy (Wyeth), Prosobee (Mead Johnson) — make up according to manufacturers' instructions

General

1   Lists of 'milk free' foods are available and should be obtained from the Department of Nutrition and Dietetics.

2   Further information about the use of milk substitutes can, usually, be obtained from

Department of Nutrition and Dietetics
Pharmacy

3   Most tube feeds and supplementary drinks are based on milk. Special milk free substitutes can be requested.

4   The following foods should be omitted in addition to those listed on p. 75:

Made up products – unless known to be milk free e.g., sausages, fish fingers, cream desserts, instant whips, creamed cereals made with milk

Chocolate (milk), toffees and fudge (boiled sweets and mints are allowed)

Packet soups and sauces – unless known to be milk free (Bovril, Oxo, Marmite, etc. are allowed)

Complan and other milk based drinks

5   In some paediatric cases a milk free diet is prescribed in conjunction with an egg free diet. If this is the case, specialist advice will be needed.

6   Calcium supplements may be required – check whether these should be given and that they have been written up by a qualified member of the medical staff.

Disorders of the Renal, Hepatic and Cardiovascular Systems

Renal replacement therapy

There are many forms of replacement therapy for non-functioning kidneys. These range from intermittent dialysis to a renal transplant. The dietary regimens are similarly varied and specific instructions should be sought in respect of individual patients.

It is unusual to restrict the protein intake once treatment has been established. The protein intake may, however, be *measured* in order to facilitate monitoring. This would still necessitate a special, therapeutic diet in most instances.

Continuous ambulatory peritoneal dialysis (CAPD) is one form of renal replacement therapy which necessitates a *high* protein intake. This is to compensate for the large amounts of protein which are lost in the dialysate. Patients on CAPD are also able to handle potassium more effectively than their counterparts on other forms of dialysis (this is due to the differing dialysis techniques). This means that their diets need not necessarily be potassium restricted.

The management of renal failure is an extremely complex subject. Further information should be sought locally from the medical and dietetic staff who are directly involved.

Dietary protein restrictions in renal failure

These vary enormously according to the type and stage of renal disease. There are many forms of renal replacement therapy and these may dictate different degrees of dietary protein modification.

Urea is one of the end products of protein metabolism and it is normally excreted by the kidneys. Urea production is directly related to dietary protein intake and serum urea levels can, therefore, be lowered by reducing the amount of protein containing foods which are eaten.

Acute renal failure

The serum urea levels tend to rise quickly as a result of an isolated event which has caused acute renal failure. The aim of dietary management is to meet the nutritional needs of the patient while simultaneously reducing the urea levels as quickly as possible.

It is important to remember that the nutritional requirements of the patient are vital. These should be met even although it may mean giving additional dialysis.

Chronic renal failure

The serum urea levels tend to rise more slowly and prophylactic dietary intervention can be usefully employed. It should be remembered that some forms of chronic renal failure are characterised by large urinary protein losses e.g., nephrotic syndrome. This protein *must* be replaced by means of an appropriate diet, otherwise the patient will start to break down his own body tissues.

Foods containing large amounts of protein

1   Meat – all types including preserved meats, tinned meats and 'made-up' meat products e.g., pies, sausages, etc.
2   Fish – all types as above
3   Eggs
4   Cheese – all types except cottage cheese although this does contain some protein (see p. 82)
5   Milk – all types including tinned and dried
Milk products including ice cream, yoghurt, milk puddings
6   Nuts – all types
7   Pulses – including peas, lentils and dried beans e.g., soy beans, kidney beans, etc.

Foods containing significant amounts of protein

1   Bread – all types
2   Cereals – all types including
Breakfast cereals
Pudding cereals e.g., semolina, rice, sago, etc.
3   Biscuits – all types
4   Flour – and all products made with flour including
Cakes
Pastries
Sauces, etc.
5   Potatoes – give average helpings only of *all* types
6   Sweets – including chocolate, toffees, fudge, liquorice

Protein exchanges

It may be advisable to substitute one type of protein containing food for another. There are two reasons for this:

1 To vary the diet.
2 To increase the energy value of the diet by including foods which can be used as 'calorie carriers' (see p. 72).

It is very important to ensure the patient takes the same total amount of protein containing foods each day.

$$\left. \begin{array}{l} \text{1 oz (25 g) lean meat} \\ \text{1}\tfrac{1}{2}\text{ oz (35 g) fish} \\ \text{1 egg} \\ \tfrac{3}{4}\text{ oz (18 g) hard cheese} \\ \tfrac{1}{5}\text{ pt (100 ml) milk} \end{array} \right\} = \text{7 g protein}$$

7 g protein = 1 meat portion

In order to modify the protein content of the diet the following information may be helpful:

1 One meat portion may be exchanged for 3 slices ordinary bread.
2 One slice ordinary bread may be exchanged for any of the following:
  Average helping breakfast cereal (not muesli)
  1 oz (25 g) flour
  3 small plain biscuits e.g., Rich Tea, Marie, etc.
  1 oz (25 g) chappatti (1 small chappatti)
  1 oz (25 g) cooked shortcrust pastry
  1$\tfrac{1}{2}$ oz (35 g) steamed sponge pudding
  1 oz (25 g) cottage cheese (1 tablespoon)
  2 oz (50 g) natural yoghurt (2 tablespoons)
  4 oz (100 g) potatoes (boiled or mashed)
  3 oz (75 g) potatoes (roast or chipped)
  1 oz (25 g) pasta (spaghetti, macaroni, etc.)

NB
1 *Remember to check possible potassium, sodium and fluid restrictions* (see pp. 85, 93 and 94).

2 *Consult the dietitian* **before** *any changes are made.*

Low protein

Aim

1 *In renal failure* – to lower the serum urea (see general note on p. 78).

2 *In hepatic failure* – to prevent the accumulation of toxic protein metabolites e.g., ammonia, which are normally broken down by the liver. An excess of these metabolites can lead to coma. As soon as liver function is restored a high protein diet is indicated.

Relevant drugs

Drug therapy is usually complex in both the above categories. It is, therefore, nearly impossible to give any guidelines and each patient's prescription should be examined individually.

Important!

1 A high calorie intake is indicated when diets are restricted in protein (see p. 84). This helps to prevent the breakdown of tissue protein which can contribute to raised serum urea levels.

NB Patients with chronic renal or chronic hepatic failure may be undernourished before their present admission (see p. 79).

2 Check whether a *sodium (salt) restriction* is required – one is often indicated in these patients. Refer to p. 86 'Foods containing large amounts of sodium'.
Refer to pp. 85–93 for further information.

3 Check whether a *fluid restriction* is required. If it is, refer to p. 93.

4 Check whether a *potassium restriction* is required – one is normally indicated in renal failure although it is not usual to restrict potassium in cases of hepatic failure.
Refer to p. 95 'Foods containing large amounts of potassium'.
Refer to pp. 94–98 for further information.

5 Make sure that the patient (and his visitors) know which foods to avoid (see pp. 95 and 97). Check the bedside locker regularly!

6 Make sure that the daily allowances of milk, bread and butter are clearly labelled and carefully stored.

Low protein: Menu modifications

This chart should be used in conjunction with the distribution chart on p. 84.

Breakfast	Cereal		*See chart* – Rice Krispies or Cornflakes only (if allowed). Milk from allowance – *see chart*
	Fruit or fruit juice	Yes	*Only* if there is no fluid or potassium restriction. Watch tomato juice (Na + content)
	Egg	Yes	*See chart*
	Bread or roll	Yes	*See chart* – white *only* if there is a potassium restriction
	Marmalade, honey or jam	Yes	
	Tea or coffee	Yes	Milk from allowance – *see chart*. **NB** No instant coffee if there is a potassium restriction
Mid-morning	Plain biscuits		*See chart* – *no* wholegrain biscuits e.g., digestive, if there is a potassium restriction
	Tea or coffee	Yes	Milk from allowance – *see chart*. **NB** No instant coffee if there is a potassium restriction
Lunch	Meat or eggs	Yes	*See chart* – *no* pastries or sauces
	Fish	Yes	*See chart* – white fish *only* if there is a sodium restriction
and	Cheese	Yes	*See chart* – *not* allowed if there is a sodium restriction
	Potatoes	Yes	*See chart* – watch cooking methods if there are sodium or potassium restrictions
Supper	Rice	Yes	*See chart* – *not* allowed if there is a fluid restriction White *only* allowed if there is a potassium restriction
	Pulses	No	Includes peas, broad beans, baked beans, etc.
	Green and root Vegetables	Yes	Small quantities only if there is a potassium restriction
	Puddings	No	Unless made with double cream and water. No ice cream
	Fresh or tinned Fruit	Yes	Watch potassium and fluid if there are restrictions. No custard unless made with double cream and water

Mid-afternoon	Plain biscuits		*See chart* – no whole grain biscuits e.g., digestive, if there is a potassium restriction
	Tea or coffee	Yes	Milk from allowance – *see chart.* No instant coffee if there is a potassium restriction
Bedtime	Plain biscuits		*See chart* – no wholegrain biscuits e.g., digestive, if there is a potassium restriction
	Milky drink	No	Plain milk may be allowed – *see chart*
	Tea or coffee	Yes	No instant coffee if there is a potassium restriction
Daily allowances	Milk Bread Plain biscuits	}	*See chart*

General

1 Butter, sugar, jam, marmalade, honey and double cream are allowed freely.

2 Special low protein bread, crispbreads and biscuits are allowed freely. They are, generally, available from either:

Department of Nutrition and Dietetics
Pharmacy
Catering Department

These products contain only very small amounts of sodium and potassium.

3 If Hycal is prescribed it has a fluid content of 125 ml per bottle which must be included in any fluid allowance. It is excessively sweet and this can be reduced by chilling.

4 If a patient is required to keep to a very restricted protein intake for a prolonged period it is advisable to monitor the haemoglobin levels regularly.

5 There are several high calorie products which are protein free and can be used in conjunction with a low protein diet (see p. 72 and Appendix V).

Table 4.4 Low protein diet – distribution

g Protein	Breakfast			Mid a.m.	Lunch and supper					Mid p.m.	Bedtime	Daily
	Cereal (1 only)	Egg	Bread (slices or roll)	Biscuits (plain) †	Meat or Fish or Cheese or Eggs	Greens & Root Veg.	Pulses e.g. Peas Broad beans Baked beans	Potato	Fruit	Biscuits (plain) †	Biscuits (plain) †	Milk
20	No	Yes	1	No	Very small at Lunch No at Supper	Large*	No	Yes	Yes	No	No	2 fl ozs (60 ml)
30	No	Yes	2	No	As above	Large*	No	Yes	Yes	2	2	7 fl ozs (200 ml)
40	No	Yes	2	2	Very small	Yes	No	Yes	Yes	2	2	10 fl ozs (300 ml)
60	No	Yes	2	2	Average	Yes	No	Yes	Yes	2	2	10 fl ozs (300 ml)

* Only if there is no potassium restriction
† 2 Plain biscuits may be exchanged for ¾ slice (¾ oz/20 g) bread

General points
a) No soup is allowed if there is a fluid restriction.
b) Sugar, butter, marmalade and jam are allowed freely.
c) If available, low protein products e.g. crispbreads may be given freely.
d) Do not give cheese and biscuits or ice-cream instead of fruit.
NB Exact quantities of meat etc are not given because this would be impractical to implement at ward level. It should be possible to obtain accurately weighed meals from the kitchen.

High protein

High protein diets are prescribed in both chronic hepatic and chronic renal failure. For further information please refer to pp. 69 and 79.

Salt and sodium restrictions – General

There is an increasing amount of evidence which demonstrates that an excessive intake of salt can be harmful to health. Many expert groups recommend that the dietary consumption of salt should be reduced. This can be done by limiting the amount of salt which is used in cooking, by restricting the foods which contain large amounts of salt and by adding less salt at table. Such a dietary modification is not classified as a therapeutic diet.

Salt and sodium restrictions – Therapeutic

1 Sodium forms part of sodium chloride (common salt). Any diet restricted in sodium should, therefore, *exclude salt*.
This means that the patient should **never** *be allowed to use the salt cellar* – make sure that it is removed from his tray.

2 There are three main levels of sodium restriction. These are:
No added salt – approximately $65-80$ mmol Na^+ per day (see p. 87)
Low salt – approximately 40 mmol Na^+ per day (see p. 89)
Low sodium – approximately 22 mmol Na^+ per day (see p. 91)

3 A low sodium diet is generally somewhat unpalatable and should not be used unless absolutely necessary.

4 Several salt substitutes (e.g., Selora, Ruthmol) are available and can be prescribed. However some are made from potassium chloride and *must never be used when a potassium restriction is indicated* e.g., renal failure.

Foods containing large amounts of sodium

These should be *avoided* if any category of salt or sodium restriction is required:

Cheese (except cottage cheese)

Bacon, ham and other preserved cold meats

Commercially prepared 'made-up' meat products e.g., meat pies, sausages, etc.

Salty fish and smoked fish e.g., kippers, smoked haddock, anchovies, etc.

Fish and meat pastes

Tinned meats, vegetables, soups and any other foods containing monosodium glutamate

Peanuts, potato crisps, etc.

Salty biscuits e.g., Ritz crackers, Tuc biscuits

Foods containing baking powder, baking soda or self-raising flour

Chocolate and cocoa or any products containing them

Ovaltine, Horlicks and other similar milk drinks, products containing any of these

Bovril, Oxo, Marmite

Lucozade, soda water

Tomato juice

Dried fruits

Spinach, celery

Ice cream

Golden syrup

Chutneys, pickles and bottled sauces (including ketchup, brown sauce and soy sauce)

No added salt
(approximately 65–80 mmol Na⁺ daily)

This is not generally classified as a special therapeutic diet and is usually ordered through the main kitchen.

Aims

1   To reduce hypertension.

2   To lower the serum sodium level.

3   To reduce oedema associated with salt and water retention.

Relevant drugs

1   Diuretics e.g., Bendrofluazide, Frusemide, Spironolactone
2   Antihypertensives e.g., Hydrallazine, Methyldopa, Captopril

Important!

1   Remember not to put a salt cellar on the patient's tray.

2   Make sure that the patient (and his visitors) know which foods to avoid (see lists on pp. 85 and 86).

3   Check with the doctor to ascertain whether or not salt substitutes e.g., Selora, Ruthmol, etc. can be used. If allowed these can, generally, be obtained from the Pharmacy.

4   Check whether or not a *fluid restriction* is required (see p. 93).

General

1   Salt is not allowed with meals but may be used sparingly during cooking.

2   Alcohol: spirits, wines and cider may be taken *with medical approval only*. Beers, lagers and stouts must be avoided.

3   Most indigestion pills and powders contain significant amounts of sodium and should *only be taken if medically prescribed*.

No added salt: Menu modifications

Breakfast	Cereal	Yes	Average helping. Milk from daily allowance
	Fruit or fruit juice	Yes	
	Egg or white fish	Yes	No smoked fish
	Bacon, sausage, etc.	No	
	Bread or roll	Yes	From daily allowance
	Butter	Yes	
	Marmalade, jam or honey	Yes	
	Tea or coffee	Yes	Milk from daily allowance
Mid morning	Plain biscuits	Yes	If used instead of bread
	Tea or coffee	Yes	With milk from daily allowance
Lunch	Meat	Yes	Plain varieties only (e.g., roast, stewed, etc.)
and	Fish	Yes	White only
Supper	Cheese	No	
	Eggs	Yes	
	Potatoes	Yes	
	Vegetables	Yes	Except spinach and celery No tinned varieties
	Pudding	Yes	(a) if milk pudding or custard – deduct milk from daily allowance (b) avoid dried fruit, golden syrup and ice cream
Mid afternoon	Bread & butter	Yes	From daily allowance
	Plain biscuits	Yes	If used as bread exchange
	Tea or coffee	Yes	With milk from daily allowance
Bedtime	Bread & butter	Yes	From daily allowance
	Plain biscuits	Yes	If used as bread exchange
	Milky drink	No	Plain milk is allowed
	Tea or coffee	Yes	With milk from daily allowance
Daily	Milk	Yes	1 pint (600 ml) only
	Bread (brown or white)	Yes	5 slices only 1 slice only can be exchanged for 2 plain biscuits or 1 soft bread roll
	Butter	Yes	1 oz only (25 g or 3 individual portions)

Low salt (approximately 40 mmol Na⁺ daily)

Aims

1 To reduce hypertension.

2 To lower the serum sodium level.

3 To reduce ascites or generalised oedema associated with salt and water retention.

Relevant drugs

1 Diuretics e.g., Bendrofluazide, Frusemide, Spironolactone
2 Antihypertensives e.g., Hydrallazine, Methyldopa, Captopril

Important!

1 Remember not to put a salt cellar on the patient's tray!

2 Make sure that the patient (and his visitors) know which foods to avoid (see lists on pp. 85 and 86).

3 Check whether a *fluid restriction* is required (see p. 93).

4 Check whether a *potassium restriction* is required. If it is not, then salt substitutes e.g., Ruthmol, Selora, etc. may be used. These can, generally, be obtained from the Pharmacy.

If a potassium restriction has been requested see pp. 94 – 97 for further information.

5 Check whether a *protein restriction* is required. If it is, refer to further information on pp. 79 – 84.

6 Make sure that the patient does not exceed his daily allowance of milk, bread and butter (see p. 91).

General

1 Alcohol – spirits, wines and cider *may only be taken with medical approval.* Beers, lagers and stouts must be avoided.

2 Most indigestion pills and powders contain significant amounts of sodium and *should only be taken if they have been medically prescribed.*

3 Creamers – non-dairy creamers (i.e. those which do not contain milk e.g., Coffeemate, Compliment, etc.) may be used occasionally if wished – check the labels carefully.

Low salt: Menu modifications

NB   *All food should be cooked without salt.*

Breakfast	Cereal	Yes	Puffed Wheat or Shredded Wheat only and milk from daily allowance
	Fruit or fruit juice	Yes	Not tomato
	Egg or white fish	Yes	No smoked fish
	Bacon, sausages	No	
	Bread or roll & butter	Yes	From daily allowance
	Marmalade, honey or jam	Yes	
	Tea or coffee	Yes	Milk from daily allowance
Mid morning	Plain biscuits	No	Unless used as bread exchange from daily allowance
	Tea or coffee	Yes	Milk from daily allowance
Lunch	Meat	Yes	Plain varieties only e.g., roast, stewed, etc.
	Fish	Yes	White only
	Eggs	Yes	
and	Cheese	No	Unless cottage cheese
	Potatoes	Yes	No salt to be sprinkled on chips, etc!
Supper	Vegetables	Yes	Except spinach and celery. No tinned varieties
	Puddings	No	Unless made with double cream and water. No ice cream
	Fruit	Yes	Fresh or tinned. No custard unless made as above
Mid afternoon	Bread & butter	Yes	From daily allowance
	Plain biscuits	No	Unless used as a bread exchange from daily allowance
	Tea or coffee	Yes	With milk from daily allowance
Bedtime	Plain biscuits	Yes	If used as a bread exchange from daily allowance
	Milky drink	No	Plain milk is allowed (from daily allowance)
	Tea or coffee	Yes	With milk from daily allowance

Daily allowances	Milk	Yes	½ pint (300 ml) only – any type of fresh milk
	Butter	Yes	½ oz (15 g) only – salt free butter is allowed freely
	Bread (white or brown)	Yes	3 slices only. 1 slice may be exchanged for 2 plain biscuits Salt free bread, salt free Ryvitas or Matzos are allowed freely

Low sodium (approximately 22 mmol Na$^+$ daily)

Aims

1 To reduce severe hypertension.

2 To lower the serum sodium level.

3 To reduce ascites or generalised oedema associated with salt and water retention.

Relevant drugs

1 Diuretics e.g., Bendrofluazide, Frusemide, Spironolactone
2 Antihypertensives e.g., Hydrallazine, Methyldopa, Captopril

Important!

1 Check that such a low sodium restriction is really necessary. This is a very unpalatable diet and should not be used for any longer than is absolutely essential.

2 Make sure that the patient (and his visitors) know which foods to avoid (see list on pp. 85–86).

3 Check whether a *fluid restriction* is required (see page 93).

4 Check whether a *potassium restriction* is required. If it is not, then salt substitutes e.g., Ruthmol, Selora, etc. may be used. These can,

Low sodium: Menu modifications

NB   *All food should be cooked without salt.*

Breakfast	Cereal	Yes	Puffed or Shredded Wheat only. Use double cream and water instead of milk
	Fruit or fruit juice	Yes	Not tomato
	Egg or white fish	Yes	No smoked fish
	Bacon, sausage, etc.	No	
	Bread or roll & butter	Yes	From daily allowance
	Marmalade, honey or jam	Yes	
	Tea or coffee	Yes	Milk from daily allowance
Mid morning	Plain biscuits	No	Unless used as bread exchange from daily allowance
	Tea or coffee	Yes	Milk from daily allowance
Lunch	Meat	Yes	Plain varieties only e.g., roast, stewed, etc.
	Fish	Yes	White only
	Eggs	Yes	
	Cheese	No	Unless cottage cheese
	Potatoes	Yes	No salt to be sprinkled on chips, etc!
	Vegetables	Yes	Except spinach and celery. No tinned varieties
Supper	Puddings	No	Unless made with double cream and water. No ice cream
Mid afternoon	Bread & butter	Yes	From daily allowance
	Plain biscuits	No	Unless used as a bread exchange from daily allowance
	Tea or coffee	Yes	Milk from daily allowance
Bedtime	Plain biscuits	No	
	Milky drink	No	
	Tea or coffee	Yes	Milk from daily allowance
Daily allowances	Milk	Yes	3fl ozs (75 ml) only. Fresh milk – any type
	Butter	No	Ordinary salted butter is not allowed. Salt free butter is allowed without restriction
	Bread (white or brown)	Yes	2 slices only. 1 slice may be exchanged for 2 plain biscuits Salt free bread, salt free Ryvitas or Matzos are allowed freely.

generally, be obtained from the Pharmacy. If a potassium restriction has been requested, see pp. 94–97 for further information.

5   Check whether a *protein restriction* is required. If it is, refer to further information on pp. 79–84.

6   Make sure that the patient does not exceed his daily allowances of milk, bread and butter (see p. 92). Make sure that these are clearly labelled and carefully stored.

General

1   Alcohol – spirits, wines and cider *may only be taken with medical approval.* Beers, lagers and stouts must be avoided.

2   Most indigestion pills and powders contain significant amounts of sodium and should only be taken if they have been medically prescribed.

3   Creamers – non-dairy creamers (i.e. those which do *not* contain milk e.g., Coffeemate, Compliment, etc.) may be used occasionally if wished – check the labels carefully. Double cream is also allowed freely.

Fluid restrictions

Monitoring fluid balance is an essential part of the management of many disease states particularly those of the renal, hepatic and cardiovascular systems. It is absolutely essential that charts are kept accurately and *all* fluid measurements are recorded frequently. The following points may be helpful:

1   All food should be served dry i.e. no gravy, syrup, etc. If these are included the quantities should be charted.

2   Foods 'made' from fluids should be avoided e.g., porridge, soup, yoghurt, ice cream, jellies, milk puddings, etc.

3   Rice *absorbs* twice its own weight in water during cooking. This *must* be deducted from the daily fluid allowance. Spaghetti,

macaroni, noodles, etc. absorb water in a similar way which should be calculated appropriately.

4   Certain fruit and vegetables contain comparatively large amounts of liquid and should be *avoided* e.g., melon, cucumber, marrow, etc.

5   Remember to measure and record the amount of fluid given with pills. Encourage the patient to take his pills with food rather than fluid if possible.

6   Puréed foods contain large quantities of liquid.

7   Check the amount of water that a cup, glass, medicine glass, ice-cube, cereal bowl, etc. hold. These will vary from unit to unit.

Low potassium

Potassium is a mineral salt which is primarily responsible for the maintenance of neuromuscular tone. Potassium balance in the body is controlled by the kidneys.

Aim

To reduce the serum level of potassium.

Relevant drugs

Calcium Resonium
Resonium A
NB   These drugs should always be given with water (not fruit juice or milk – see p. 95).

Important!

1   Many of these patients may be on dialysis and should know which foods to avoid. However, it is prudent to remind them (and their visitors) – see p. 95.

2   Check whether a *fluid restriction* is required (see p. 93).

3   Check whether a *protein restriction* is required (see p. 79 for 'Foods containing large amounts of protein' and pp. 78–84 for further information).

4   Check whether a *sodium (salt) restriction* is required (see p. 86 for 'Foods containing large amounts of sodium' and pp. 87–93 for further information).

5 *Never* use salt substitutes e.g., Selora, Ruthmol, etc.

6 Check the patient's locker regularly (see below) especially in respect of extra fresh fruit and chocolates.

Foods containing large amounts of potassium

The following foods must *never* be taken because of their high potassium content:

1 Instant coffee (e.g., Nescafé, Maxwell House, Gold Blend, etc.) and instant tea (e.g., Lemsip, Lift, etc.). Percolated coffee, filtered coffee, leaf tea and tea bags are allowed

2 Chocolate and any products containing chocolate

3 Dried fruits e.g., raisins, sultanas, prunes, dates, etc. and any products containing dried fruit
Dried vegetables e.g., peas, onions, peppers, etc. and any products containing them e.g., packet soup mixes

4 Nuts – all types including ground almonds and desiccated coconut and any products containing them e.g., marzipan, peanut butter, wholefood bars (Jordans, Prewetts, etc.)

5 Wholegrain cereals including
Breakfast cereals e.g., Weetabix, Shredded Wheat, All Bran
Wholemeal and other similar breads
Brown rice
Wholegrain biscuits and crackers e.g., digestive, Ryvita, etc.
NB These may be allowed however under careful medical/dietetic supervision.

6 Salt substitutes e.g., Ruthmol, Selora, etc.

7 Concentrated fruit drinks e.g., Ribena, canned or frozen juice

8 Malted milk drinks e.g., Horlicks, Ovaltine, etc.

9 Bovril and Oxo

10 Molasses and black treacle

11 All beers, stouts, lagers and cider

12 Fruit squashes (mineral waters are permitted freely *provided* that there is no fluid or sodium restriction)

13 Curry powder – this can be allowed as an exchange; consult the dietitian for further information.

Low potassium: Menu modifications

Breakfast	Cereal	Yes	Cornflakes, Rice Krispies or Sugar Puffs only. No wholegrain cereals are allowed. Milk from allowance
	Fruit	No	Unless taken from daily allowance
	Fruit juice	No	
	Egg, bacon, fish, etc.	Yes	*Check* any other restrictions e.g., protein, sodium, etc.
	Tomatoes or mushrooms	No	
	Bread or roll & butter		White only
	Marmalade, jam or honey	Yes	
	Tea or coffee	Yes	*No* instant coffee – milk from allowance
Mid morning	Bread, butter and jam	Yes	White bread only
	Plain biscuits	Yes	*No* wholegrain biscuits e.g., digestive
	Tea or coffee	Yes	*No* instant coffee – milk from allowance
Lunch	Meat, fish, cheese or eggs	Yes	*No* sauces. *Check* any other restrictions e.g., protein, sodium, etc.
	Potatoes	Yes	*Small* portions only. Avoid chips, roast and baked potatoes if possible
and	Pulses	No	Includes lentils, peas and dried beans
	Green vegetables and salad vegetables	Yes	Small portions only – no vegetables from list on pp. 95 and 97
Supper	Pudding	Yes	Except those containing fruits listed on p. 95 and 97. **NB** Any custard, milk pudding, yoghurt, etc. would have to be included in the daily milk allowance. Check any other restrictions e.g., protein, sodium, etc.
Mid afternoon	Bread, butter and jam	Yes	White bread only
	Plain biscuits	Yes	*No* wholegrain biscuits e.g., digestives
	Tea or coffee	Yes	*No* instant coffee – milk from allowance

Bedtime	Plain biscuits	Yes	*No* wholegrain biscuits e.g., digestives
	Milky drink	No	Plain milk from daily allowance
	Tea or coffee	Yes	*No* instant coffee – milk from allowance
Daily	Milk	Yes	½ pint (300 ml) only – any type of fresh milk
	Fruit	Yes	3 servings only – either fresh, stewed or tinned. *No* dried fruit is allowed

General

1 If the patient is receiving dialysis treatment he should not, generally, eat foods which contain large amounts of potassium while on dialysis (see p. 95).

2 *No* toffees or fudge are allowed (in addition to items on p. 95). Boiled sweets, mints, Turkish Delight (no chocolate coating) and chewing gum are permitted.

3 Alcohol – clear spirits e.g., gin, whisky, brandy, etc. *are allowed only after medical approval* has been given. Beers, lagers and stouts must never be taken. Sherry and wine are allowed occasionally (*after medical consent has been obtained*).

4 *No* fruit squashes, etc. are allowed (see also p. 95). Fizzy mineral waters are permitted.

5 In addition to the list on p. 95 the following foods should also be *avoided*
Mushrooms, tomatoes, spinach and baked beans
Fresh apricots, peaches and damsons, no extra bananas or oranges
Potato crisps

6 If the patient has to maintain a potassium restriction for a prolonged period it may be advisable to monitor his intake of Vitamin C and supplement it with ascorbic acid tablets if necessary.

High potassium

This is not normally considered to be a therapeutic diet and would be ordered through the main kitchen.

Potassium is a mineral salt which is widely distributed in food. The potassium content of foods is significantly reduced by prolonged contact with water. If a high intake of potassium is required the following groups of foods should be *included* in the daily meal plan:

1 Dried foods e.g., dried fruits and products containing them, instant coffee powders, etc.

2 Vegetables which are cooked quickly e.g., chips, sautéed vegetables, etc.

3 Concentrated fruit drinks, e.g., Ribena or other blackcurrant cordial, canned fruit juices.

For further information about foods which contain large amounts of potassium, please refer to p. 95.

Low cholesterol

Cholesterol is a complex fat-like compound and is widely distributed in animal tissues. The cholesterol content of the diet can often be reduced by lowering the overall intake of fat containing foods.

Aim

To lower the serum cholesterol levels and associated complications by

1 Reducing the intake of dietary fats

2 Replacing some of the 'saturated' fats in the diet (usually of animal origin) by 'polyunsaturated' fats and oils (usually of vegetable origin)

Low cholesterol: Menu modifications

Breakfast	Cereal	Yes	No muesli. Milk from allowance
	Fruit or fruit juice	Yes	
	Egg	No	Unless taken from weekly allowance
	Bacon	Yes	Lean only – grilled
	Fish	Yes	
	Bread or roll	Yes	
	Butter		Scraping only – use polyunsaturated margarine if possible
	Marmalade, honey jam	Yes	
	Tea or coffee	Yes	Milk from allowance
Mid morning	Plain biscuits	No	
	Tea or coffee	Yes	Milk from allowance
Lunch	Lean meat or fish	Yes	No pastries or sauces
	Eggs or hard cheese	No	Cottage cheese is allowed
and	Potatoes	Yes	Not creamed; either plain boiled *or* fried or roasted in oil (watch calories)
	Pasta and rice	Yes	No butter or fat unless poly-unsaturated
	Vegetables	Yes	All types – do not add butter
Supper	Pudding	Yes	Yoghurt, fruit or jelly only. Milk puddings are allowed only if skimmed milk is used from allowance
Mid afternoon	Bread, butter and jam	Yes	Scraping butter only or polyunsaturated margarine
	Plain biscuits	No	
	Tea or coffee	Yes	Milk from allowance
Bedtime	Plain biscuits	No	
	Milky drink	No	Unless skimmed milk
	Tea or coffee	Yes	Milk from allowance
Daily	Milk	Yes	½ pint (300 ml) skimmed milk or 2 oz skimmed milk powder
	Polyunsaturated margarine	Yes	Not more than 1 oz (25 g)
Weekly	Egg yolks	3	Egg whites are allowed freely

Relevant drugs

Clofibrate (Atromid-S)
Cholestyramine (Questran)
Dextrothyroxine (Choloxin)
Nicotinic acid

Important!

1 Dairy products e.g., eggs, butter, milk and cheese contain large amounts of cholesterol. These should either be *omitted* (and replaced with other products) or restricted as follows:

Eggs – not more than 3 egg yolks each week (egg whites are allowed freely).

Butter – replace with a margarine which is labelled 'High in Polyunsaturated Fats' or with a low fat spread.

Milk – use skimmed milk or skimmed milk powder.
Cheese – only cottage cheese is permitted. All other cheeses should be excluded.

2 Other fat containing foods should be monitored e.g.
Meat should be lean with all visible fat removed (offal such as liver is not allowed).
Fried foods should be restricted if the patient is obese.
All fat used in cooking should be polyunsaturated.

3 *Weight* – many patients are able to lower their serum cholesterol level by reducing their weight. Check that a *calorie restriction* is not required (see p. 51 for further information about high calorie foods).

General

1 Many foods contain 'hidden' fats. These are generally animal fats which contain significant amounts of cholesterol. The following foods should be *avoided*:

Cakes, biscuits and pastries of any type
Chocolates, toffees and fudge (all other sweets are allowed)
Ovaltine, Horlicks and similar beverages (tea, coffee, fruit juices, fruit squashes and mineral waters are permitted)
Cream soups (clear soups are allowed)
Nuts (all types)
Made-up meat dishes e.g., sausages, pâté, etc.

2   Encourage the patient to take some exercise if this is practical.

3   Alcohol is not permitted unless medical consent has been obtained beforehand.

Miscellaneous Diets

Low calcium

Calcium is the mineral directly concerned with the formation of teeth and bones. It is an important constituent of the blood and plays a major role in the clotting mechanism and enzyme activity. It is also involved in the regulation of muscle tone.

Aim

To lower the serum level of calcium

Short-term — for specific diagnostic tests
Long-term for conservative management of specific pathological conditions e.g., renal calculi.

Relevant drugs

Calcitonin
Sodium cellulose phosphate
Phosphate Sandoz
NB   Diarrhoea may occur as a consequence of using these drugs.

Important!

1   Only 2 litres of tap water should be allowed each day for *all* purposes. Distilled water should be used if additional water is needed.

2   If the diet has been prescribed in the short-term for a specific test, it is prudent to order it for longer than it is actually required.

3   Milk and milk products *are not allowed* (see pp. 75–7).
100% wholemeal bread *only* should be used (ordinary brown bread contains more calcium and is not suitable).

4   Additional Vitamin D should *not* be given unless it is specifically prescribed.

5   Check the patient's locker regularly to ensure that no unsuitable foods are brought in. Visitors may bring in boiled sweets, fruit squashes and apples.

General

1   Any cups of tea, coffee, etc. and any drinks (including water taken with tablets) should be deducted from the daily allowance of tap water.

2   The following foods should be *avoided*:

White flour and any products made with white flour including bread, biscuits, cakes, pastries, sauces, etc.

Milk and any products except butter made from milk or containing milk e.g., cheese, ice cream, yoghurt, cream soups, milk puddings, etc. This includes milk based drinks e.g., Complan, Ovaltine, Horlicks, etc.

Eggs

Fish with bones and shell fish e.g., kippers, herrings, sardines, pilchards, whitebait, eels, etc. This includes fish pastes.

Vegetables – the following should be avoided: broccoli, spinach, spring greens, spring onions, turnip tops and watercress.
All others are allowed freely.

Fruit – the following should be avoided: blackberries, blackcurrants, olives and rhubarb, all dried fruit e.g., dates, prunes, raisins, sultanas, etc.

Oranges are allowed *in moderation only*.

All others are allowed freely.

Nuts (all types)

Chocolates, toffees and *fudge* of all types. Boiled sweets are allowed.

Low calcium: Menu modifications

Breakfast	Cereal	Yes	Cornflakes or Rice Krispies only – no milk
	Fruit or fruit juice	Yes	
	Bacon, fish, tomatoes	Yes	White fish only
	Egg	No	
	Bread or roll	Yes	Wholemeal only
	Butter, marmalade, honey, etc.	Yes	
	Tea or coffee	Yes	No milk – water from allowance
Mid morning	Bread or roll	Yes	Wholemeal only
	Butter and jam	Yes	
	Plain biscuits	No	
	Tea or coffee	Yes	No milk – water from allowance
Lunch	Meat or fish	Yes	White fish only
	Cheese or eggs	No	
	Potatoes or rice	Yes	No mashed or creamed potatoes
and	Vegetables	Yes	See 'General' comments
	Pudding	No	
Supper	Fruit	Yes	See 'General' comments
	Cheese and biscuits	No	
	Tea or Coffee	Yes	No milk – water from allowance
Mid afternoon	Bread or roll	Yes	Wholemeal only
	Butter and jam	Yes	
	Plain biscuits	No	
	Tea or coffee	Yes	No milk – water from allowance
Bedtime	Plain biscuits	No	
	Milky drink	No	
	Tea or coffee	Yes	No milk – water from allowance
Daily	Milk	No	A non-dairy, non-filled creamer may be used instead of milk – check the label
			Locasol is a calcium free milk product which can usually be obtained from Dept. of Nutrition and Dietetics Catering Pharmacy
	Butter or margarine	Yes	Allowed freely
	Tap water	Yes	2 litres only

Low purine

Purines are complex substances formed as a result of the metabolism of proteins. They are broken down into uric acid.

Aims

1   To lower the serum levels of uric acid and reduce the amount of uric acid crystal formation (a common cause of renal calculi, etc.).

2   To measure the excretion of purines from non-dietary sources. This is sometimes used as a confirmatory diagnostic test.

Relevant drugs
Allopurinol
Probenecid
Sulphinpyrazone

Important!

1   Drug therapy can be very effective; not all patients on uric acid lowering drugs are on low purine diets.

2   This is not a 'weighed' diet – the intake of purine is only lowered.

3   If the diet has been prescribed in the short-term for a specific test, it is prudent to order it for slightly longer than it is actually required.

General

1   Only *one* serving of meat or fish is allowed each day.

2   Alcohol is usually *forbidden* on this type of diet. It should only be included after medical consultation.

3   The following foods *must be completely excluded*:

Offal including liver and kidneys
Gravies and meat extracts e.g., Bovril, Oxo, etc. This includes soups made from these products.
Sardines
Wholegrain cereals and any products containing them e.g., wholemeal bread, digestive biscuits, wholemeal crispbreads, porridge and other wholegrain breakfast cereals

Low purine: Menu modifications

Breakfast	Cereal with milk	Yes	Cornflakes or Rice Krispies only
	Fruit or fruit juice	Yes	
	Bacon, fish, etc.	No	
	Bread or roll	Yes	White only
	Butter and marmalade or honey	Yes	
	Tea or coffee and milk	Yes	
Mid morning	Bread or roll	Yes	White only
	Butter and jam	Yes	
	Plain biscuits	Yes	No digestives or other wholegrain biscuits.
	Tea or coffee & milk	Yes	
Lunch	Meat or fish	Yes	*Once* daily only. *No* gravy. *No* sardines
	Cheese or egg	Yes	
	Potatoes or rice	Yes	
and	Vegetables	Yes	See 'General' comments
	Puddings	Yes	*No* wholegrain flour, etc.
Supper	Fruit	Yes	See 'General' comments
	Cheese and biscuits	Yes	*No* wholegrain crispbreads
	Tea or coffee & milk	Yes	
Mid afternoon	Bread or roll	Yes	White only
	Butter and jam	Yes	
	Plain biscuits	Yes	No digestive or wholegrain varieties
	Tea or coffee & milk	Yes	
Bedtime	Plain biscuits	Yes	No digestive or wholegrain varieties
	Milky drink	Yes	Nothing chocolate based Plain milk is allowed freely
	Tea or coffee & milk	Yes	

Vegetables — cauliflowers, mushrooms, peas, spinach and all dried vegetables including lentils and dried beans.

All other vegetables are allowed freely.

Fruit — all dried fruit e.g., dates, prunes, raisins, sultanas, etc.

All other fruits are allowed freely.

Nuts (all types)

Chocolate (all types and varieties including chocolate based milk drinks)

Gelatin free (collagen free)

Collagen is the connective tissue in the body and forms the intercellular 'cement'. It is a protein based compound.

Aims

1   To reduce the serum levels of hydroxyproline caused by the breakdown of collagen.

2   To assess the rate of muscle protein breakdown and thereby assess nutritional status.

Relevant drugs

These will vary according to the diagnosis of individual patients and should be considered on that basis.

Important!

1   This diet is generally prescribed on a short-term basis for a specific test. It is prudent to order it for longer than it is actually required.

2   Make sure that the patient knows which foods should be avoided. Check his locker regularly during the test period to ensure that no unsuitable foods are brought in.

General

The following foods *must be excluded completely* from the diet:

1   Meat and poultry – all types including sausages, hamburgers, pastes, etc. Products made exclusively from textured vegetable protein are allowed.

2   Fish – all types including sardines, anchovies, pastes, etc.

3   Soups and sauces with meat or fish bases.

4   Puddings – no jellies, ice creams, mousses, whips, etc.
Milk puddings, plain yoghurt, fruit and pastry dishes are allowed.

5   Preserves – no jams or marmalades. Honey and golden syrup are allowed.
Chutneys and pickles should be avoided.

Gelatin (collagen) free: Menu modifications

Breakfast	Cereal with milk	Yes	Any type
	Fruit or fruit juice	Yes	
	Egg	Yes	
	Bacon, fish etc	No	
	Bread or roll & butter	Yes	
	Marmalade or jam	No	Honey is allowed
	Tea or coffee & milk	Yes	
Mid morning	Bread or roll & butter	Yes	
	Jam	No	Honey is allowed
	Plain biscuits	Yes	
	Tea or coffee & milk	Yes	
Lunch	Meat or fish	No	Unless a textured vegetable protein product is used
	Cheese or eggs	Yes	
	Potatoes or rice	Yes	
	Vegetables (all types)	Yes	
and	Puddings	Yes	Fruits, milk puddings, plain sponges, plain yoghurt
		No	Jellies, ice cream, mousses or anything containing jam
Supper	Cheese & biscuits	Yes	No processed cheese
	Tea or coffee & milk	Yes	
Mid afternoon	Bread or roll & butter	Yes	
	Jam	No	Honey is allowed
	Plain biscuits	Yes	
	Tea or coffee & milk	Yes	
Bedtime	Plain biscuits	Yes	
	Milky drink	Yes	
	Tea or coffee & milk	Yes	

6   Sweets – no pastilles, toffees, fruit gums or soft sweets, e.g., Turkish Delight, are allowed.
Boiled sweets and plain mints are allowed freely.

Metabolic and/or research studies

These are extremely accurate studies involving the exact measurements of dietary intakes which are then compared with excretion rates in respect of particularly defined nutrients.

Metabolic balance studies are usually carried out

1   To confirm a diagnosis
2   To assess the effect of a particular form of treatment e.g., drug trials.

Units undertaking this type of work will usually have a specifically designated Metabolic Unit which will have its own kitchen. A dietitian is often attached to such a unit and she will supervise any studies which are implemented.

It is inappropriate to undertake metabolic studies without having access to specialist facilities. If these facilities do exist then individual protocols will be available in respect of various tests.

It is extremely important that everyone who is involved in this type of study (including the patient) is aware of

1   The purpose of the study
2   The length of the study
3   The protocol for the particular study
4   The importance of meticulous weighing and recording
5   The importance of adhering rigidly to the prescribed guidelines

---

MAOI Therapy

Mono-amine oxidase inhibitors are used for a wide group of patients and this is one group of drugs for which there are specific nutritional recommendations which must be followed. The limitations which are required can, usually, be achieved by minor modifications to the main menu.

Aims

1   To prevent the occurrence of migraine type headaches.

2   To prevent possible collapse or other adverse side effects caused by the interaction of MAOI drugs and specific foods.

Relevant drugs

Mono-amine oxidase inhibitors (MAOIs) e.g., Phenelzine, Iproniazid, Isocarboxazid, Tranylcypromine

Important!

The following foods *must be omitted* completely from the diet:

1 Cheese – all types
2 Bovril, Oxo and other meat extracts*
3 Marmite and other yeast extracts*
4 Wines, beers and other alcohol
5 Pickled herrings
6 Broad bean *pods*

* **NB** Remember to check that gravies are not made with these products.

In addition some centres recommend that
Yoghurt
Flavoured textured vegetable protein products
are also *omitted* from the diet.

5
Special Formula Feeding

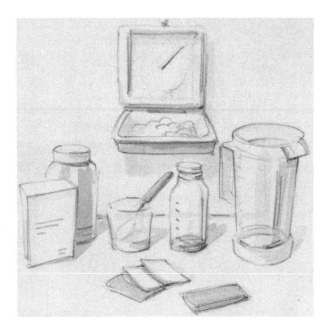

Fig. 5.1 Formulae diets

Elemental formulae

These are also called 'No Residue' diets and were initially evolved in the course of research leading up to the first manned space flights in the 1960's. Nutrition is presented in a pre-digested, easily absorbed mixture of proteins, carbohydrates and fats. The following preparations are formulated in this way:

Vivonex: Standard
               HN   } Norwich-Eaton Laboratories

Elemental 028 Scientific Hospital Supplies

Aims

1   To reduce faecal content to a minimum in order to
Prepare a patient for surgery
Control acute malabsorption e.g., Cröhns disease, ulcerative colitis, short bowel syndrome, etc.
Achieve initial control with ileostomies and colostomies

2   To improve nutritional status when normal food cannot be tolerated. Sometimes this is the preferred form of feeding when IV nutrition is being considered in the following instances:
Pre- and post-operatively
To help close fistulae
When the available absorptive area is reduced e.g., intestinal resection. (There should be a minimum of 100 cm of small intestine remaining in order to absorb the elemental diet.)

Important!

1   *Follow the mixing instructions meticulously.*
These products are not very pleasant but they are quite acceptable if they are mixed correctly (also see p. 112). They should be sipped slowly. (They can also be given nasogastrically.)

2   Explain to the patient that he will not be receiving normal meals. *It is extremely important that he does not eat or drink anything else other than* **clear fluids only** *while on this diet* (see p. 36). Make sure visitors are aware of this.

3   Remember to warn the patient that his faecal volume will be greatly reduced – there may be only one motion each week.

4   These preparations are expensive and should only be used as specifically prescribed. They should never be used to supplement ordinary food.

5   These preparations are *not* suitable for infants and children.

6   Make sure that you have all the information you need to simplify the use of these formulae. Further details can usually be obtained from:
Department of Nutrition and Dietetics
Pharmacy

General

1   Maintain a positive attitude towards the patient about taking these preparations. A great deal of encouragement will probably be needed.

2   Elemental diets are packed in powder form. They can be reconstituted in a variety of ways by using different flavours, temperatures (e.g., soups) and textures (e.g., jellies). Try and introduce as much variation as possible.

3   If the diet is to be served as a drink (rather than as a soup) *make sure that it is chilled thoroughly.*

4   Make sure that the mixture is *not boiled* if it is to be served as a soup.

5   Elemental diets should be taken slowly i.e. one glass should be sipped slowly over an hour.

6   The unpleasant taste can often be reduced by taking the diet through a straw.

7   Only make up the amount which will be needed for one 'meal'. Discard any feed which is left over after 24 hours.

Minimal residue formulae

Recent research has shown that proteins may be absorbed more effectively if they are not presented as pure amino acids. The following preparations contain di-peptides as well as amino acids:

Flexical (Mead Johnson)
MCT Pepdite (Scientific Hospital Supplies)
Nutranel (Roussel Laboratories)
Pepdite (Scientific Hospital Supplies)
Peptisorbon (Merck)
Salvipeptid (MCP Pharmaceuticals)
Triosorbon (Merck)

The indications for the use and administration of these products are exactly the same as those for Elemental Diets (pp. 110–112).

Special milk formulae (paediatrics)

These specially designed products are intended for use in conjunction with a specifically diagnosed abnormality which prevents a baby from taking the normal proprietary baby milk preparations.

Important!

1 Always check the label on the tin to make sure that it contains *exactly* what you think it does.

2 Further information about particular products and their uses can usually be obtained from

Department of Nutrition and Dietetics
Pharmacy

Other important considerations

1 A product should be prescribed for a specific condition and other, similar products may not be as suitable. If any changes are necessary, check with the medical staff first.

2 Make sure that the formula being used is 'in date'. The expiry date is displayed on the container – after which the formula should never be used.

3 Follow the mixing instructions meticulously and make sure that the formula is diluted correctly.

4 Discard any excess made-up formula after 12 hours.

5 Make sure that the parents know exactly how the formula should be used and how they can obtain further supplies.

6 These products must be medically prescribed and the dietitian should be closely involved when a regimen is implemented.

NB The issue of standard (proprietary) baby milk products is *usually* controlled by the Catering Department.

Table 5.5 Special paediatric milk substitutes

Product	Protein			Fat			Carbohydrate						
	Milk	Soya	Other	MCT	Other	Glucose	Galactose	Sucrose	Lactose	Fructose	Corn syrup	Starch
Formula 'S'		Soy protein isolate + Methionine			Vegetable Oil	✓						
+Galactomin 17	Washed casein				Coconut + Maize	Liquid						
+MCT (1)-Milk	Washed casein			✓	Liquid							
Nutramigen	Enzyme hydrolysed casein *			✓	Corn			✓				✓
Portagen	Sodium caseinate			✓	Corn			✓			Solids	

Table 5.5 (*Contd.*)

Product	Protein			Fat		Carbohydrate						
	Milk	Soya	Other	MCT	Other	Glucose	Galactose	Sucrose	Lactose	Fructose	Corn syrup	Starch
Pregestimil	Enzyme hydrolysed casein *			✓	Corn						Solids	✓
Prosobee (powder)		Soy protein isolate + Methionine			Soya			✓			Solids	
Prosobee (liquid)		Soy protein isolate + Methionine			Soya + Coconut			✓			Solids	
Wysoy		Soy protein isolate + Methionine			Coconut + Soya + Safflower			✓				

* Charcoal treated to reduce allergenicity
+ These are not complete foods and require vitamin/mineral supplementation

Special paediatric milk substitutes

The following list is only intended as a guide and gives an
indication of the uses of the formulae which are prescribed more
commonly.

Product	Manufacturer	Clinical indications for use
Formula S*	Cow and Gate	1 Intolerance of cow's milk protein (casein) or lactose. 2 Galactosaemia
Galactomin 17†*	Cow and Gate	1 Lactose intolerance 2 Galactosaemia 3 Galactokinase deficiency
MCT (1) – Milk†*	Cow and Gate	Fat malabsorption: 1 Pancreatic disease 2 Hepatobiliary disease (including obstructive jaundice) 3 Cystic fibrosis 4 Gastrectomy 5 Intestinal resection 6 Intestinal lymphangiectasis
Nutramigen**	Mead Johnson	1 Intolerance of cow's milk protein (casein) or lactose 2 Persistent diarrhoea, vomiting and/or colic 3 Post-operative recovery from intestinal surgery 4 Galactosaemia 5 Galactokinase deficiency 6 Maintenance of nutrition during test on elimination diets
Portagen	Mead Johnson	1 Fat malabsorption: Biliary disease Chronic liver disease 2 Cystic fibrosis 3 Following intestinal surgery 4 Lactose intolerance
Pregestimil*	Mead Johnson	1 Fat malabsorption 2 Disaccharidase deficiency or lactose deficiency 3 Cystic fibrosis 4 Following intestinal surgery 5 Chronic diarrhoea

Product	Manufacturer	Clinical Indications for use
Prosobee (liquid or powder)	Mead Johnson	1 Milk allergy 2 Galactosaemia 3 Galactokinase deficiency 4 Lactose intolerance
Wysoy	Wyeth	1 Milk intolerance or allergy 2 Lactose intolerance 3 Galactosaemia 4 Galactokinase deficiency

† These products are *not* complete foods and require vitamin and mineral supplementation.
* These products are sucrose free.
** Recommended only for use in infants over 3 months old.
NB Comminuted chicken meat (Cow and Gate) should not be used as a replacement for milk. It is carbohydrate and milk-protein (casein) free and is, therefore, useful in the management of disorders involving intolerances of these substances.
An outline of the main components of each formulation is given on pp. 114–115.

6

Nutritional Management of the Grossly Compromised Patient

Body composition in health and disease

The human body is composed of water, minerals including sodium and potassium and organic compounds, protein, carbohydrates and fats which are integrated in various tissues in differing proportions. The structural unit in all tissues is the cell. The individual organs of the body differ from each other because their cells have a unique structure and specialised biochemical pathways. Water is present throughout the body. The organic compounds are almost entirely intracellular or in the plasma, while electrolytes are both intra- and extracellular, but in different proportions. This difference is maintained by the cell membranes by an energy consuming mechanism – the sodium pump.

In order to survive, the body requires a continuous supply of energy. The principal fuels are carbohydrate and fat.

Metabolic pathways are the routes by which essential biochemical changes are induced by enzymes, converting nutrients into energy and the other materials necessary for life. These pathways may be complex. The Krebs cycle or citric acid cycle operates in cell mitochondria and this pathway is responsible for 90% of the energy derived from carbohydrate and fats. Intermediate products in the cycle are used as substrates in the synthesis of steroids, protein, haem and nucleotides. The overall reaction is the complex oxidation of compounds which enter the cycle providing carbon dioxide and energy.

The human body will transform chemical energy to produce energy for mechanical, synthetic and electrical work. In disease states the accumulation of chemicals may interfere with the Krebs cycle activity as for example in uraemic patients when haemoglobin formation is impeded by the suppression of the activity of several enzymes in the synthetic pathway from succinyl-CoA.

The principal components which make up body weight are body water, bone, lean body mass and fat.

| | Cell | Extracellular fluid | |
	Intracellular fluid	Interstitial fluid	Intravascular fluid
Na^+	8	143	140
K^+	140	4	4
Cl^-	8	115	105
HCO_3^+	14	30	25
Ca^{2+}	1.1	1.2	2.3
Mg^{2+}	15	1.2	1
PO_4^{2-}	80	2	1

Fig. 6.1   Electrolyte concentrations in body fluids (mmol/l)

Body water

Total body water accounts for about 53 % of total body weight. The largest component is the intracellular volume, which makes up 30 % of body weight. This volume is critical and minor changes in cell hydration can result in illness and even death. The other component, the extracellular volume, is sub-divided into fluid in the vascular system and interstitial fluid between the blood vessels and the cells. Changes in extracellular volume are consistent with life and indeed they may change markedly in disease states such as cardiac failure. The electrolyte concentrations vary in the body compartments (see Fig. 6.1).

Bone

The skeleton provides a framework in which the muscles can act and it also provides protection for vital organs such as the rib-cage protecting the heart. Bone is a specialised connective tissue consisting of collagen fibres, polysaccharides and extracellular water. Its unique property of hardness is due to mineral crystals, calcium and phosphorous salts and calcium hydroxide. In addition, bone contains sodium, magnesium, fluoride, citrate and carbonate.

Chronic malnutrition in children results in delayed maturation of bone and consequent small stature, as the essential elements of bone growth may not be present in sufficient quantity. In adults, inadequate diet.

The lean body mass

This is the body engine and performs the fundamental processes
needed to sustain life; resting metabolic expenditure is related to
the size of the lean body mass. It is the work-performing and
energy-consuming component of the body, the cells which are
hydrated and rich in potassium and nitrogen. Preservation of the
lean body mass is the prime nutritional priority and the aim of
feeding a wasted patient is to restore lost lean body mass. This is a
variable quantity of body weight.

Nitrogen is assimilated into protein by the various combinations
of amino acids. The amino acids found in human protein are listed
below. Some amino acids cannot be synthesised by the body and
must be contained in the diet — these are the essential amino acids.
In some disease states arginine and histidine cannot be synthesised
in sufficient quantities and thus become essential. The amino acids
are linked together in different sequences to form different
proteins. Amino acids may be synthesised into proteins or used in
other ways, for example to provide carbohydrate by the process of

Table 6.1 Amino acids present in man

Alanine	Lysine
Arginine	Methionine
Aspartic acid	Phenylalanine
Cysteïne/Cystine	Proline
Glutamic acid	Serine
Glycine	Threonine
Histidine	Tryptophan
Isoleucine	Tyrosine
Leucine	Valine

NB Also citrulline and ornithine are
involved in urea production.

Table 6.2 Essential amino acids for adults

In Health	Leucine	Phenylalanine
	Isoleucine	Threonine
	Lysine	Tryptophan
	Methionine	Valine
Additionally with trauma or disease	Arginine	
	Histidine	

Table 6.3 Where amino acids are utilised

Liver	Muscle	Both
Arginine	Isoleucine	Aspartic acid
Histidine	Leucine	Glutamine
Methionine	Valine	Glutamic acid
Lysine		Glycine
Phenylalanine		Proline
Threonine		
Tryptophan		

gluconeogenesis where the amino acid is broken down by chemical reactions. The nitrogen part of the amino acid is excreted from the body in the urine. If total nitrogen excretion exceeds intake, this results in a negative nitrogen balance indicating loss of lean body mass.

The lean body mass has two principal components, muscle and viscera. Skeletal muscle may account for up to 40% of the total body weight of an adult. Among the viscera the liver is the principal organ of metabolism of many dietary components. It is also a storage organ for iron, copper, trace elements and Vitamins A, B and B_{12}. Energy is stored in the liver as glycogen. Indeed so complex are the liver functions that it may be likened to a major industrial company producing many different chemicals and products.

Fat

Fat is essentially the individual's portable energy store. Fat is used to provide energy when there is inadequate intake or absorption of

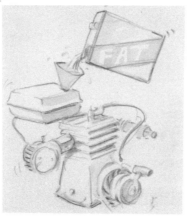

Fig. 6.2 The lean body mass functions like an engine

energy. Some vitamins (A, D, E & K) are soluble only in fat, and body fat is also involved in maintenance of body temperature. Fats are mixtures of different triglycerides (which are esters of fatty acids and glycerol). Phospholipids are another lipid component, while sterols, of which cholesterol is the most important, are involved in the transport of fatty acids. Three fatty acids, linoleic, linolenic and arachidonic are required for growth and cell membrane stability and are known as essential fatty acids.

Starvation

An uninjured and otherwise healthy man can withstand deprivation of all nutrients for comparatively long periods of time — up to 90 days. The exception to this is water. Lack of food can occur in many situations such as famine, but in clinical practice it is usually associated with disease when there has been either decreased intake or increased loss of protein, calories, and vitamins or as a direct consequence of the disease process. Early in starvation there is a reduction in the weight of the viscera including the liver, pancreas and gastrointestinal tract. Following the selective loss of liver protein in early starvation the liver becomes adapted for gluconeogenesis (production of carbohydrate from protein and fatty acid oxidation). In the gastrointestinal tract there is a loss of intestinal mucosa and digestive enzymes with a slowing of the regeneration of the mucosa. There is also a reduction in the absorptive surface of the small bowel and decreased synthesis of pancreatic enzymes, all of which result in the gastrointestinal tract becoming intolerant of food with associated refeeding problems.

As protein breakdown gradually decreases in more prolonged starvation, the circulating amino acid pool in the blood is reduced because the amino acid uptake is minimal and the turnover of proteins is decreased. Certain key organs, particularly the central nervous system, red and white blood cells, fibroblasts and the adrenal glands, usually require glucose as the principal energy source. Thus the provision of glucose during starvation is essential.

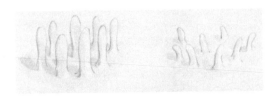

Fig. 6.3 Loss of absorptive area of small bowel in starvation (left, normal; right, starvation)

Liver is the principal site of gluconeogenesis with the amino acids being provided from the skeletal muscle. The kidney is also a site of gluconeogenesis. In early starvation 90 % of gluconeogenesis is carried out in the liver and 10 % in the kidney but this is modified later to 45 % and 55 % respectively. One kilogram of fat provides 8,100 calories and in starvation fat becomes an increasingly important energy source. After three days of starvation both muscle and liver increase the utilisation of fat. This is as a result of increasing the pool of free fatty acids and the muscle will then derive up to 90 % of its calorie requirement from their oxidation. The main products of fatty acid oxidation are ketone bodies. By using ketone bodies as a principal source of energy the demand for glucose is reduced and there is a decrease in gluconeogenesis thus preserving muscle.

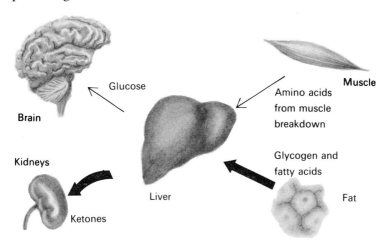

Brain

Glucose

Kidneys

Ketones

Liver

Amino acids
from muscle
breakdown

Muscle

Glycogen and
fatty acids

Fat

Fig. 6.4 Metabolic changes seen in starvation

Starvation results in a progressive and relentless loss of body weight. Progressive weight loss of more than 35–45 % is life threatening. The weight loss is rapid in the early stages and then decreases to reach a plateau. During the first ten days there is an 8–9 g/day loss of nitrogen in otherwise healthy men, which reflects loss of muscle, while after ten days this is reduced to 2–4 g/day as the obligatory glucose requiring organs such as the brain adapt to the oxidation of ketones (derived from the fat stores) as an energy source.

In prolonged but otherwise uncomplicated starvation 10–15 % of the calories are derived from protein while the remainder is produced from fat. A paradoxical situation arises whereby the need to obtain energy to maintain vital body functions results in muscle loss to provide some of that energy; this loss means the body engine is slowly being reduced in size. At first, the body faced with severe food loss turns all its metabolic activities to the single aim of survival. Body temperature is maintained but there is gradual loss of lean body mass and fat to provide energy and to protect against electrolyte changes, cell membrane changes and vitamin and mineral deficiencies. The patient becomes increasingly weak and apathetic and loses weight, and there is a gradual inability to maintain vital body functions.

Trauma

There are also nutritional changes chiefly characterised by progressive weight loss following trauma such as a surgical operation, burns, and road accidents. As early as 1927 it was observed that following the fracture of a bone there was increased nitrogen loss in the urine and a negative nitrogen balance far greater than that which would have been expected due to starvation alone. In starvation the chemical messengers such as insulin, thyroid hormones and the adrenal hormones (the chemical compounds which influence chemical reactions) show little change and the net result is an attempt to minimise protein loss in the face of inadequate intake. After injury the endocrine secretions show changes in their levels and there is a protein loss; both changes are greater than would occur with starvation alone. The mechanism of activation of the endocrine response is not fully understood, but blood loss, tissue damage, serum electrolyte changes, pain and fear are all potent stimuli. This change, known as the metabolic

Table 6.4 Typical daily post-operative nitrogen loss

	Nitrogen loss (g)	Muscle loss (g)
Herniotomy	3	80
Appendicectomy	6	200
Cholecystectomy	12	320
Fractured femur	15	400
Partial gastrectomy	15	400
Oesophagectomy	90	2500
Peritonitis	18	570
Sepsis	23	730

500 g = 1.1 lb

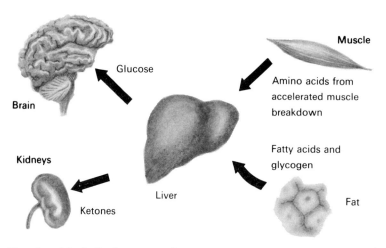

Fig. 6.5 Metabolic changes seen in trauma

response to trauma, may be quantitated by nitrogen balance studies. In general, the magnitude and duration of the response depends upon the severity of the injury and the presence of complications. The quantitation for various surgical operations is given in Table 6.4. Fat utilisation is greatly increased (by up to five- or six-fold) in the post-trauma period and there is also an increase in resting energy consumption.

Sepsis

In septic patients energy consumption is elevated, fat utilisation may be sharply reduced and continued protein breakdown provides the calories needed. The end result is further depletion of the lean body mass.

In the clinical situation the greatest loss of protein is seen in the initially wasted patient who requires major surgery and who then develops septic complications. This is a potentially lethal combination, remembering that the ideal is the preservation of the body engine or lean body mass.

Nutritional assessment

Malnutrition, be it due to starvation, the effect of severe un-complicated surgery, the effect of sepsis, or a combination of all three, results in a loss of lean body mass and body fat, both reflected as a loss of body weight. In addition, there may be associated water, electrolyte, vitamin and trace element imbalances which must also be measured. Acute weight loss of more than 40 % is nearly always fatal, while varying degrees of weight loss, irrespective of the cause, are associated with both an increased death rate and increased rate of complications if surgery is undertaken. These complications include:

Delayed wound healing
Decreased rate of union of bone fractures
Decreased resistance to infection because of immunological depression

Table 6.5   Clinical causes of starvation in hospital patients

Central Nervous System	Cerebrovascular accident
	Head injury
	Cerebral oedema
	Drug overdose
Lack of Food Intake	Anorexia nervosa
	Change in sensation of taste
	Oral or neck surgery
	Oral infections
	Chronic breathlessness
Inability to Swallow	Bulbar palsy
	Myasthaenia gravis
	Blockage of oesophagus
Failure to Absorb Foodstuffs	Gastric lesions
	Coeliac disease
	Pancreatic disease
	Renal disease
	Liver disease
	Inflammatory bowel disease
	Intestinal diverticulae
	Intestinal fistulae
	Bowel resection
	Malignant disease
	Radio or chemotherapy
	Burns
	Multiple trauma
	Chronic cardiac valve disease
	Drug/nutrient interactions
Increased Requirements	Sepsis
	Burns
	Multiple trauma
	Acute renal failure

Disordered coagulation
Reduced enzyme synthesis
Decreased tolerance to radiotherapy and chemotherapy
Prolonged convalescence after surgery because of increased weakness
Altered drug metabolism. This is changed by reduction in enzyme synthesis, thus affecting metabolic processes and changes in protein binding of drugs. Loss of minerals and trace elements such as zinc and magnesium also interfere with drug metabolism, and Vitamin C is critical, particularly in the elderly for proper drug metabolism.
Altered nutrient metabolism

When to start nutritional support

The decision whether a patient needs nutritional support is critical and should be made on the basis of clinical acumen that the patient may be wasted together with simple bedside measurements of nutritional status. The calculation of the percentage weight loss over time gives an initial indication of the degree of weight loss, and the dietary history may give an indication of specific deficiencies. No single abnormal parameter in the tests described should be used in isolation to identify malnutrition, but rather a combination of at least three measurements should be used. These should be simple and give results which are easily understood. A frequently used method to identify nutritional depletion is:

1 Recent weight loss in excess of 10% of weight in health.
2 Serum albumin level less than 32 g/l.
3 Reduction in arm circumference below 85% of the standard value.

General

The most important factor in the nutritional assessment of an individual patient is to be aware that a patient might be wasted. Several tests depend on constant observers for accuracy. This can be ensured by:

1 **Dietary history.** Specific questions about past and present nutritional intake can be most valuable in detecting deficiencies.

2 **Weighing the patient.** Comparison of his actual weight with an ideal weight taken from height and weight tables gives an approximate guide to the severity of nutritional depletion.

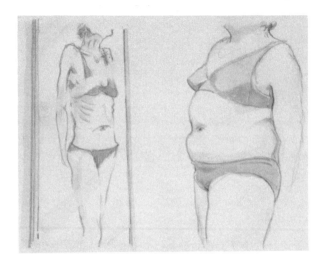

Fig. 6.6   Is the patient as well-nourished as you think?

Remember that oedema and obesity can mask the depletion of lean body mass. The percentage weight loss can then be calculated:

$$\text{Percentage weight loss} = \frac{\text{usual weight} - \text{actual weight} \times 100}{\text{usual weight}}$$

The interpretation of the percentage weight loss with time is shown in Table 6.6.

Table 6.6   Evaluation of percentage weight change

Time	Significant loss	Severe loss
1 Week	1–2	> 2
1 Month	5	> 5
3 Months	7.5	> 7.5
6 Months	10	> 10

3   **The mid-upper arm circumference in the non-dominant arm.** This measures the mass of muscle and fat of the upper arm and is a reflection of the body stores. Reduction to less than 85 % of standard adult values is associated with a significant mortality and complication rate after surgery (see Table 6.7).

Table 6.7 Mid-arm circumference values in adults
The measurement is to be made in the middle of the non-dominant arm

	Male (cm)	Female (cm)
Standard	29.3	28.5
90 % of standard	26.3	25.7
80 % of standard	23.4	22.8
70 % of standard	20.5	20.0
60 % of standard	17.6	17.1

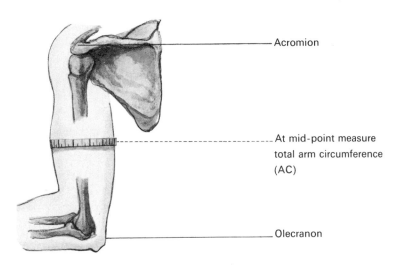

Acromion

At mid-point measure total arm circumference (AC)

Olecranon

Fig. 6.7 Method of measuring mid-arm circumference

Protein stores

This is the principal nutritional component for measuring the lean body mass, that active, energy-consuming, work-producing component which is the engine of the body. The absolute size of the muscle mass is most easily measured by:

1 **24 hour urinary creatinine estimation.** In skeletal muscle creatine is irreversibly converted to creatinine at a constant rate. Measurement of urinary creatinine in 24 hours would thus give an estimate of the skeletal mass. Three consecutive 24 urinary

collections should be performed. The nurse must ensure no urine is lost and that all the urine passed over 24 hours is collected. The values obtained are compared with those in well nourished subjects of the same height. The values of 60–80 % of normal indicate moderate malnutrition and muscle loss, while values less than 60 % indicate severe depletion.

2 **Dynamometry.** Muscle hand grip strength using a dynamometer is a good index of malnutrition showing that muscle strength falls progressively with loss of muscle. This is a simple bedside measurement. It is measured by squeezing the instrument as hard as possible on three occasions using the non-dominant arm. Values 85 % of normal or less in relation to the age and sex of the patient indicates malnutrition (see Table 6.8).

Table 6.8   Grip strength – non-dominant arm

	Normal (kg)	85 % of normal (kg)
18–69 years		
Male	40	34
Female	27.5	23
70–79 years		
Male	32.5	27.5
Female	25	21
Over 80 years		
Male	22.5	19
Female	20.0	17

3 **Skin fold caliper measurements.** The absolute size of the lean body mass may be measured simply at the bedside by calculating the total amount of body fat and subtracting that from the body weight. This is valid if the patient shows no clinical signs of being dehydrated or waterlogged. The skin fold thickness taken at four sites, mid-biceps, mid-triceps, subscapular and supra-iliac may be determined to calculate the percentage of body weight as fat. The weight of the lean body mass in kilograms, may be obtained by subtracting body fat from total body weight.

4 **Nitrogen balance.** Nitrogen balance is widely used as a method for measuring daily improvement or deterioration in the size of the body nitrogen pool, i.e. the lean body mass.

Nitrogen balance = nitrogen intake − nitrogen loss

This is calculated from intake and loss from all sources. The nurse has a vital role to play in helping with this vital estimation as a daily measure of improvement or deterioration by ensuring that fluids from all sites (urine, fistulae, nasogastric loss and faeces) are collected methodically and completely. Uncertainty about the completeness of the collections can change the calculated balance. If more nitrogen is retained than lost, tissue synthesis − anabolism − is taking place, but if loss is greater then tissue breakdown or catabolism is occurring. A balance of one gram of nitrogen indicates a change of 6.25 grams of protein or 30 grams of muscle tissue.

5 **Visceral protein.** The visceral (as opposed to the skeletal component of the lean body mass) may also be measured. This is a measure of liver protein synthesis. Assuming the patient is not dehydrated or overhydrated, a serum albumin concentration between 30 g/l to 21 g/l may suggest moderate malnutrition, and values less than 21 g/l, severe malnutrition. Serum transferrin is also a measure of visceral protein synthesis. Its normal range is 20− 30 g/l. A serum concentration of 1.0−1.50 g/l may suggest moderate malnutrition and values less than 1.0 g/l severe malnutrition. False elevations of serum transferrin levels occur in patients with chronic blood loss and blood transfusion.

Fat stores

Measurements of body fat are an estimate of the body's energy stores. The simplest measurement is to use skin fold calipers and measure triceps skin fold thickness on the non-dominant arm (Table 6.9). The interpretation is shown in the table. Significant

Table 6.9	Triceps	skinfold	thickness
	values in adults		
		Male (mm)	Female (mm)
Standard		12.5	16.5
90% of standard		11.3	14.9
80% of standard		10.0	13.2
70% of standard		8.8	11.6
60% of standard		7.5	9.0

loss of fat occurs with values below 10 mm for men and 13 mm for women.

Immune status

Adequate nutrition is essential to maintain a normal immune response as a defence mechanism against infection. In malnutrition there may be a reduction in the peripheral lymphocyte count, $800-1200/ml^3$ indicates moderate protein calorie malnutrition, less than $800/ml^3$ indicates severe depletion.

Minerals

In water electrolytes dissociate into ions which have either a positive or negative charge.

Sodium. This is the main extracellular electrolyte and it affects water distribution throughout the body so that if sodium is lost, water is also lost and vice versa. Sodium in the body is carefully controlled by the kidney. A low serum sodium is found in water excess (over hydration), malnutrition, vomiting, diarrhoea, gastrointestinal fistula loss and renal disease. High levels are usually associated with excess salt intake or dehydration. Normal serum sodium levels are 137–144 mmol/l.

Potassium. This is the main intracellular electrolyte, the concentration in the cell being about thirty times greater than in the blood. The high intracellular potassium and low sodium concentrations are maintained by an active process in the cell membrane known as the sodium pump. The effectiveness of the pump may decline in starvation, or after injury or sepsis, thus allowing more sodium into the cell while potassium is lost. An intracellular deficit of potassium can, therefore, occur with no change in serum levels. Potassium is needed with nitrogen for protein synthesis in the cell, as well as for intracellular enzyme activity and muscle contraction. Raised serum levels are found with cell damage, acidosis and renal failure. Low levels occur in gross malnutrition, with potassium free intravenous infusions and there is increased loss with vomiting, diarrhoea, the use of diuretics and gastrointestinal fistula loss. Normal serum levels are 3.5–4.8 mmol/l.

Magnesium. This is also mainly an intracellular electrolyte and is closely involved as a co-factor in enzyme function and is a component of bone. Low levels may be found in malabsorption, prolonged nasogastric suction and prolonged intravenous infusion and fistulae losses. Normal serum levels are 0.7 – 1.0 mmol/l.

Calcium. Most calcium is present in bone, but it is also found in the plasma and the cell. Calcium is absorbed from the lower small intestine and excretion is controlled chiefly by the kidney. Two hormones, parathormone and calcitonin, have a major effect upon calcium metabolism. Low levels may be particularly found in malabsorption and pancreatitis and produce excessive nerve and muscle excitability – tetany. Raised levels are associated with increased parathormone levels, bone disease and renal failure. The normal serum calcium is from 2.2 – 2.6 mmol/l.

Chloride. This is the principal electrolyte with a negative charge. Chloride changes usually follow those of sodium but in some circumstances bicarbonate may also change. Normal serum levels are 96 – 108 mmol/l.

Bicarbonate. Bicarbonate is a buffer regulating excess acidity in the body. Raised levels are found with excess infusion of plasma or bicarbonate solutions or with prolonged 'drip and suck' regimes. Low levels are seen in shock, respiratory failure, diabetes, starvation and renal failure. Normal serum levels are 23 – 28 mmol/l.

Phosphate. Phosphates have many functions as enzymes associated with fat metabolism and in the formation of the skeleton. Plasma levels rise in renal failure and fall in some endocrine diseases, such as hyperparathyroidism and in prolonged intravenous feeding. Normal plasma levels are 0.6 – 1.5 mmol/l.

Vitamin and trace elements status

Vitamins. The daily requirements of vitamins vary greatly. In the body's engine the vitamins are the 'spark plugs' without which the energy cannot be properly used. Vitamins are organic substances required for the maintenance of life, even though they may only be present in small amounts. There are two types, water soluble (B & C) and fat soluble (A, D, E & K). The fat soluble vitamins are absorbed from the intestine with dietary fats and stored in the body while the water soluble vitamins are rarely stored in the body.

A good nutritional history is essential to indicate any deficiency in vitamins before they are manifest clinically. There are two types of tests for vitamin status: blood concentrations or the measurement of an enzyme in which the vitamin is a co-factor. Blood levels of Vitamins A, C (ascorbic acid), B_{12} and folate reflect recent dietary intake, while white cell Vitamin C and red cell folate values indicate whole body stores. Vitamin B1 (thiamine) status and Vitamin B_6 (pyridoxin) status are measured by red cell enzyme activity. Coagulation factors are Vitamin K dependent and a prolonged prothrombin time is indicative of Vitamin K depletion.

The requirements of water soluble vitamins are especially increased with disease.

Low folate values occur with:
  Epileptic therapy
  Methotrexate treatment of cancer
  Excess alcohol intake

Vitamin B6 concentrations are *decreased* with:
  Oral contraceptives
  Isoniazid anti-tuberculosis therapy

Vitamin B_{12} deficiency occurs with oral hypoglycaemic agents.

Vitamin C depletion is found in:
  Smokers
  Association with aspirin and barbiturate therapy
  Post-operative patients

Vitamin K deficiency may occur with broad spectrum antibiotic therapy. A combination of low Vitamin A, B_6 and C values is known to reduce the immune response to infection.

Trace elements. The body contains approximately 40 elements which are present in varying amounts. Those in which the concentrations are approximately 100 parts/million in adults are known as the trace elements. Up to 15 of these are known to be required for health and knowledge is expanding rapidly. Some trace elements are involved in cell membrane function and others in enzyme function. Indeed about one-third of all enzymes which modulate the chemical processes related to nutrition are dependent upon trace elements. Trace element deficiencies are usually associated with gross malnutrition, and in prolonged artificial feeding, especially parenteral nutrition, it becomes important to supplement the trace metals. In gross deficiency clinical manifestations may be found.

Zinc depletion. This is associated with anaemia, dermatitis, diarrhoea and impaired wound healing.
Copper with iron resistant anaemia and osteoporosis.
Chromium with glucose intolerance and peripheral neuropathy.
Selenium with bone disease.

The principles of nutritional management

The fundamental principle of management is that if a patient is able to eat and the gastrointestinal tract is functioning, then oral or enteral feeding is always the method of choice. Parenteral feeding is appropriate if these criteria are not met. Irrespective of the method employed the basic requirements of nutritional replacement are:

1 To maintain the circulation.
2 To achieve water and electrolyte replacement and balance.
3 To replace lost lean body mass and thus to restore the body engine to full power again.

Recent studies suggest that up to one-half of all patients in hospital may be malnourished and indeed some may leave worse than they arrived, having missed meals because of investigations, the stress of surgery, unappetising food and many other minor causes all contributing to loss of weight. Awareness by the doctor or nurse that a patient may be malnourished or at risk of becoming so is the key to success and the common clinical conditions where nutritional support may be needed are listed in Table 6.10 and on p. 15.

To feed a patient by whatever route many nutrients must be supplied including nitrogen, energy, water, electrolytes, vitamins, trace elements. The requirements for these may change daily. The many nutrients needed are interlinked and must be supplied constantly if the metabolic functions of the body are to be fully maintained with resulting tissue synthesis. The problem for the clinician achieving this is rather like that of a juggler having to keep about twenty different objects in the air at the same time – no mean accomplishment.

A monitoring system must be used during a feeding regimen to determine whether the nutrient balance is being maintained (see Appendix VIII, Table 1). This is a comprehensive list of both simple and sophisticated tests, but it is essential to a successful

Table 6.10   The principal clinical indications for nutritional support
(See also Table 6.5)

Pre-operative Nutritional Depletion
Post-operative Complications:
  a   Ileus more than 4 days
  b   Sepsis
  c   Fistula formation
  d   Failure to achieve required intake within 5 days
Intestinal Fistula
Massive Bowel Resection
Management of:
  a   Pancreatitis
  b   Malabsorption Syndromes
  c   Ulcerative Colitis
  d   Radiation Enteritis
  e   Pyloric Stenosis
Anorexia Nervosa
Intractible Vomiting
Maxillofacial Trauma
Traumatic Coma
Multiple Trauma
Burns
Malignant Disease
Renal Failure
Liver Disease
Cardiac Valve Disease
Chronic Breathlessness

outcome. Complications may ensue despite this producing clinical symptoms during the feeding regimen. The commonest complications and the means of correcting them are given in Appendix IX, Table 1. The nurse is a critical figure in the prevention of problems by ensuring the accurate collection of all losses and the conscientious and accurate charting of all intake and output.

Requirements

Nitrogen. Nitrogen has to be supplied in any oral or parenteral feeding regimen in the correct amount, correct form and with other nutrients. In enteral diets whole protein is probably best, but some diets known as 'elemental' diets have nitrogen as amino acids, and dipeptide mixtures are also available. Enteral diets (containing

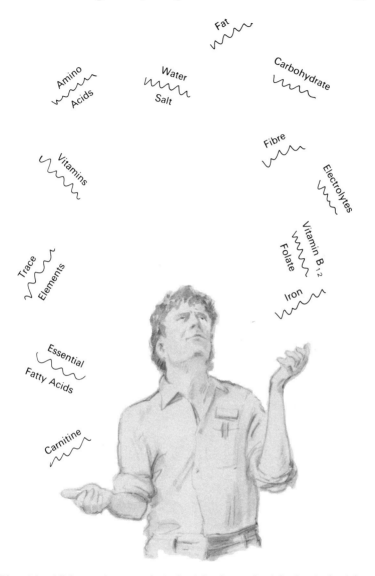

Fig. 6.8 All the nutrients must be in the right place at the right time in the right amounts

all the required nutrients) approximate more to the normal situation by producing a feeding response in the human intestine, hence stimulating absorption. In intravenous feeding solutions, nitrogen is given as amino acids (see Appendix VII, Table 2). Sufficient amounts of the essential amino acids (leucine, isoleucine, valine, methionine, phenylalanine, lysine, tryptophan and threonine, and in disease, arginine and histidine) must be present. Daily nitrogen balance studies give the best indication of total nitrogen requirements.

Energy. This is usually provided in a mixed form as glucose and fat. There is certainly a close relationship between the energy supplied and nitrogen utilisation. The energy requirement of the starving patient is comparatively low, a calorie: nitrogen ratio of about 200 calories per gram of nitrogen. This ratio changes in the post-operative or septic patient. Ideally the requirement should be calculated for the individual patient. Other constituents of the diet such as potassium, phosphate and zinc also influence the efficiency of nitrogen utilisation. In addition, nitrogen assimilation with the same energy intake is much improved if the patient can be mobilised.

Electrolytes and minerals. Electrolyte imbalances must be prevented or corrected and this is done by regular biochemical monitoring. Approximate daily requirements are known and are shown in Appendix VII, Table 4. Low serum phosphate levels may occur particularly with intravenous feeding, while approximately 6 mmol of potassium are required for each gram of nitrogen in order for it to be incorporated into protein. Iron supplements may be required for haemoglobin synthesis and trace elements are given in long-term feeding although the precise daily requirements for many remain unknown.

Levels of zinc, manganese and copper must be monitored in the blood and supplements may be especially required in patients on long-term parenteral feeding.

Vitamins. Vitamin deficiencies can occur quickly. Although vitamins are essential for the efficient utilisation of foodstuffs, the precise requirements still remain to be fully worked out. The recommended daily intake and the commercially available intravenous solutions together with their constituents are shown in Appendix VII, Table 3.

There is a multiplicity of oral vitamin preparations for patients being fed enterally. Each differs in vitamin content and dosage and so careful checking is needed to ensure the patient is receiving what he requires from these enteral vitamin preparations. It is important that the vitamins not given in the oral or intravenous multivitamin preparations – Vitamins K, B_{12}, folic acid and D – are supplied by whatever route is appropriate (folate 5mg twice weekly IV and Vitamin B$_{12}$ 250 µg weekly IM or IV).

To meet all the many and changing requirements of the patient is a difficult task. There are many potential hazards and difficulties. The success of enteral and parenteral nutrition depends upon good organisation, accurate record keeping and co-operation between many different people. The recent trend to the formation of specialist nutrition teams is invaluable in improving the standard of care. The individual disciplines mentioned below are usually represented on specialist nutrition teams:

1   *Nursing staff.* The nurses are very important as they are expected to maintain accurate delivery of nutrients, correct records and, in the case of parenteral feeding, scrupulous asepsis. A specialist nursing sister is invaluable for supervision and teaching.

2   *Dietitian.* The dietitian has a unique role in dietary asssessment; her skills help to prevent illogical distinctions being made between 'food' and 'enteral feeding'.

The dietitian is the link between:

Patient's needs and expectations of food
Nutritional assessment/requirement
Medical prescription
Nurse's care of patient
Cook's provision of appropriate food

3   *Pharmacist.* The role of the pharmacist is in parenteral feeding and is important not only in making additives and mixtures professionally and in ideal conditions, but in his ability to advise about compatibility of different mixtures of nutrients and their storage potential. Recently he has acquired a major role in the preparation of 3 litre bags for parenteral feeding (see Appendix VIII, 5).

4   *Laboratory staff (Biochemists & Bacteriologists).* They provide a laboratory analysis of specimens sent so that fundamental measurements can be made, such as those of nitrogen balance. Bacteriologists should carry out strict surveys of aseptic technique in the management of problems of patients being fed parenterally, who develop unexplained swings in temperature.

5   *Clinician.* It is advantageous if a clinician with a special interest in nutrition co-ordinates the team, as this provides both a focus for the team and a final arbiter. This is usually a consultant surgeon or physician.

7
Oral or Enteral Feeding

The most common method used to feed patients is for food to be introduced into the gastrointestinal tract then absorbed through the bowel into the blood stream, resulting eventually in tissue synthesis. Once an individual patient needs special feeding and the nutrients required have been decided upon then nutrition should be provided in the simplest, cheapest way which is at the same time the most acceptable to the patient.

Oral feeding

Ordinary food is the first choice, providing the patient has a reasonable appetite, can swallow and has a functioning gastrointestinal tract. Although a normal diet may suffice, many factors may reduce both appetite and enjoyment of food (see p. 15). Disturbances of taste – dysgeusia – may be the result of many causes, some of which are listed in Table 7.1. Any inflammation of the gums must be corrected. Apathy and anorexia may occur if there is a fever, or in inflammatory bowel disease, acute hepatitis, carcinoma of the pancreas and congestive heart failure. A low blood sodium, high blood calcium, digoxin therapy and the use of sedatives also compromise successful oral feeding.

Table 7.1   Causes of changes in taste

Loss of smell
Damage to nerves
Endocrine insufficiency
    a   thyroid
    b   adrenal
Low serum copper or zinc
Uraemia
Drugs
    a   carbimazole
    b   tranquillisers
    c   lincomycin tetracycline
    d   penicillamine

Tube feeding

When a patient cannot tolerate oral feeding or is unable to swallow, then feeding through a tube should be considered. The tube may be passed through the nose into the stomach – a nasogastric tube – or directly inserted through the anterior abdominal wall into the upper bowel – an enterostomy; as it is usually inserted into the jejunum, it is then called a jejunostomy.

Nasogastric feeding. A recent major advance has been the use of fine bore polyvinyl or polyurethane nasogastric tubes, rather than the larger Ryle's tube. These finer tubes are more comfortable, do not cause stricture formation and may be left in place for longer periods. If there is a narrowing in the oesophagus before feeding then the fine bore tube may be passed into the stomach using a fibre-optic endoscope.

Jejunostomy feeding. The insertion of a fine bore catheter the skin and into the jejunum as a definitive surgical procedure will allow the upper gastrointestinal tract to be by-passed and nutrients infused directly into the small bowel where absorption takes place. The risk of pulmonary aspiration or the increased incidence of chest infections associated with the use of nasogastric tubes is reduced and patients find it more acceptable. However, the technique of fashioning a jejunostomy is a surgical procedure with the risks associated with surgery and leakage may result in skin irritation around the stoma.

There is a wide choice of products available for enteral feeding (see Appendix V, 4). Administration of an enteral feed either via a nasogastric tube or a jejunostomy should be carefully supervised, and the rate of infusion monitored.

In starvation or during parenteral nutrition when nutrients are not in direct contact with the bowel lining, the absorptive capacity of the bowel declines. There are two causes; firstly, the height of the villi or finger-like folds of bowel which greatly increase the absorptive surface area decline with a consequent decreased absorption. Secondly, the enzymes in the bowel lining involved in the digestive process also decrease, further impairing absorption. These changes occur within three days of the onset of starvation and result in less efficient absorption of food from the bowel. This also affects the institution of enteral feeding.

There are potentially numerous complications, the most common being listed in the table below. An awareness of possible complications is the critical factor in their prevention.

Table 7.2 Complications of tube feeding

Feeding tube insertion
  a   misplacement
  b   withdrawal

Bowel side-effects
  a   abdominal distension or pain
  b   diarrhoea

Regurgitation and inhalation into the lungs

Metabolic
  a   high blood sugar levels
  b   low potassium, calcium and phosphate blood levels
  c   low zinc and folate levels

Changes in liver function

Accidental intravenous administration of enteric feeds

Bacterial contamination of the feed

Complications associated with enteral nutrition

Passage of the fine bore tube into the stomach may be confirmed by X-ray, showing the tube in the stomach and not in a bronchus.

Regurgitation and inhalation may be avoided by initially ensuring adequate gastric emptying and careful regulation of the infusion rate, perhaps using a pump. Bowel disturbances may occur in up to one-quarter of all patients. The commonest side effect is abdominal pain, usually a colic associated with abdominal distension. A slow introduction to the full feeding regimen over three days or so will reduce the incidence. Diarrhoea may be a particularly troublesome problem; the rate of infusion, adjusting the osmolar load, the use of broad spectrum antibiotics, a high fat or sodium content of the feed and the lactose content are all associated causes.

Metabolic complications are prevented ideally by careful biochemical monitoring during feeding. Hyperglycaemia, a high blood sugar, may be the result of excessive glucose intake or the patient's difficulty in utilising the sugar particularly in the immediately post-operative period or if the patient is septic. Electrolyte disturbances, particularly a low serum potassium, calcium, phosphate, zinc and magnesium, may occur and must be corrected. Changes in liver function tests during enteral feeding are sometimes found, the cause is unknown but they are usually transitory and return to normal at the end of feeding.

Tube feeding

There may be occasions when it is not possible to feed a patient adequately using the preferred oral route. There are four main reasons for this:

1 *Physical:*
Obstruction or restriction of the mouth and throat e.g., oesophageal carcinoma, facial trauma, wired jaws.
Acute inflammation e.g., following radiotherapy, dental disease.
Loss of swallowing reflex e.g., cerebrovascular accident, Guillain-Barré syndrome.

2 *Psychological:*
Dislike of hospital conditions and feeding routines (see p. 15)
Anorexia nervosa
General loss of appetite e.g., elderly, chronic depressed states.

3 *Long standing pathological conditions leading to depressed appetite:*
Carcinoma (particularly the GI tract)
Inflammatory illness which may be exacerbated by certain foods e.g., Cröhn's disease, ulcerative colitis, peptic ulcer.
Chronic systemic failure e.g., renal or hepatic failure, chronic cardiac valve disease.

4 *Increased requirement for nutrition:* including
Sepsis
Catabolic disease
Protein-losing conditions
    Burns
    Enterocutaneous fistulae
    Nephrotic syndrome
    Major trauma

The results of an inadequate nutritional intake have been clearly documented in current medical and nursing literature and have been referred to i.1 greater detail on p. 118. *Awareness* of the possibility of undernutrition (for whatever reason) is a vital factor in the subsequent management of the hospital patient and cannot be overemphasised. Attention to nutritional status should be considered to be an integral part of the medical management of the patient.

Once it has been decided that the patient is not achieving the required intake of food it is vitally important to initiate alternative feeding methods at the earliest opportunity. No patient should be allowed to go without food/nutrition in hospital unless this has been prescribed specifically in connection with particular medical or surgical procedures.

There are many ways in which normal food can be supplemented using the oral route and these should be considered first (see p. 34).

It may not always be feasible to use these methods – in which case supplementation of the oral intake can be effected by means of a tube feed. This can be administered for a varying length of time – usually overnight or continuously over the 24 hour period. The composition of the supplementary feed will be calculated to make up the difference which exists between the patient's normal daily diet and his daily nutritional requirement. It is worth noting that this type of feeding can stimulate the appetite and that the patient may, apparently spontaneously, be able to eat greater quantities of food.

Unfortunately many patients will not be able to benefit from this type of feeding programme. It then becomes necessary to consider *total enteral nutrition* (i.e. delivering all the patient's required nutrition directly into the GI tract). There are several methods of achieving this and these should all be evaluated carefully before considering the alternative of *total parenteral nutrition* (intravenous feeding, see p. 165). It is important to remember that this text should only be considered as a guide to enteral nutrition and must be read in conjunction with any local policies and procedures which exist for the feeding of patients by this method. It is advisable to involve a dietitian – who has specialised knowledge of the subject – at the earliest opportunity.

There are three main routes by which food can be introduced enterally:

1 Nasogastric
2 Nasoduodenal
3 Feeding stoma e.g., gastrostomy or jejunostomy (see p. 141)

The points which follow regarding feeding methods, equipment, solutions and monitoring apply equally to all three routes except where stated to the contrary. All the considerations which are mentioned should be determined by the condition and requirements of each individual patient.

Method

Continuous gravity drip feeding

In many cases this is the method of choice. Feeding is by means of a constant infusion which is economical in terms of nursing time.

There is less risk of diarrhoea due to the sudden delivery of a nutrient load to the stomach or small intestine and the administration rate can be closely monitored and readily modified with minimal discomfort to the patient.

Continuous feeding using an enteral infusion pump

There are some occasions when it may be necessary to administer the feed very slowly or very accurately. Commercial enteral pumps are available for this purpose and are easy to use. They require special modification to the giving sets (see p. 150) but are convenient and generally reliable. It should *not* be necessary to use a pump of this nature for routine feeding procedures.

Intermittent feeding (Gravity drip or Pump assisted)

Various categories of patients are particularly restless and confused e.g., alcoholic liver disease, elderly, etc. This can cause problems if a solution is administered continuously. In these cases intermittent feeding regimens can be initiated. This involves continuous feeding for a short period followed by a rest for a similar length of time e.g., 2 hours feeding followed by 2 hours rest over a 12–24 hour period. This means that the position of the distal end of the tube can be checked regularly. It is also more acceptable physiologically.

Bolus feeding

This is a more traditional method of feeding patients whereby a proportion of the total intake is poured down the feeding tube by a nurse either using a large syringe and allowing the feed to flow through it, or by pouring the solution directly from a jug. There is an increased likelihood of diarrhoea due to gastric 'dumping' (see above) and it can be difficult to modify the administration rate conveniently. There is, however, much closer supervision of the patient during the actual feeding process. This is an important consideration if there is any likelihood of a restless patient inadvertently dislodging a feeding tube.

Whichever method of feeding is chosen two points must be remembered:

1   Check the local nursing procedure regarding intubation technique.

2   Always ensure that the distal tip of the tube is correctly sited. This should be undertaken regularly during feeding and can be done in one of three ways:

X-ray. This is the most reliable method and should be used if at all possible when the tube is initially sited (most feeding tubes currently on the market are either radio-opaque or have a metal tip).

Aspiration. Using a 3-way tap and a 2–10 ml syringe withdraw some of the gastric contents and check both the acidity and the fact that the stomach is emptying properly (see Appendix VI, 1).

Auscultation. This is a useful means of checking the position of the tube once feeding has commenced. This is done by injecting air down the tube into the stomach and by listening for a 'burbling' sound through a stethoscope placed over the epigastrium.

NB   Aspiration and auscultation are not appropriate for checking the position of a nasoduodenal tube or a feeding stoma tube. X-ray checks should be carried out in these instances.

Never commence enteral feeding until the position of the feeding tube has been confirmed. Check the position of the feeding tube regularly.

Equipment

This can be conveniently divided into the categories of
Tubes
Giving sets
Reservoirs
Enteral feeding pumps

Tubes

A bewildering variety of feeding tubes is currently available. If the choice of tube is left to the nursing staff the following points (apart from the cost) should be considered:

1   Length
This varies from 80 cm to 210 cm. Before deciding the appropriate length of tube the method of feeding must be clarified (see p. 144). It is inadvisable for instance, to use a long nasoduodenal tube if nasogastric feeding is required. Alternatively, there may be

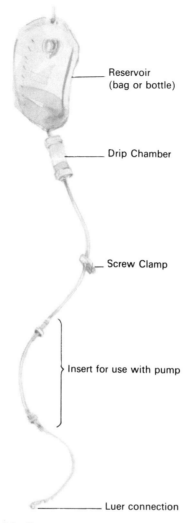

Reservoir
(bag or bottle)

Drip Chamber

Screw Clamp

Insert for use with pump

Luer connection

Fig. 7.1 Standard feeding system

instances when a greater length of tubing is required near the patient's nose (e.g., bolus feeding regimens). Many tubes have marked distances down their length to facilitate correct positioning.

2 Diameter

Again this varies widely – from French Gauge 4–20. Both the internal and external diameter of the tube should be considered because some tubes are made with thicker walls than others. It is not always necessary to use an extremely fine bore tube but the selected tube should have as small a diameter as is consistent with prescribed nursing care. This will, usually, be a French Gauge 6–8. As the width of the feeding tube is increased, so is its rigidity and it will become much less comfortable for the patient to tolerate. This is particularly important if the patient is being encouraged to eat orally with a feeding tube *in situ*. The width of the tube is also a prime consideration when intubating the elderly, in cases of oesophageal constriction or when long-term enteral feeding is planned.

The feeding tube should not generally be used for the introduction of any other substances into the patient. However, *if* no alternative route is available drugs should be given as elixirs if possible and any tablets should be crushed to a fine powder. The tube should *always* be flushed through with water after the administration of any drugs.

NB   Nasogastric formulae feeding tubes should not be confused with nasogastric aspiration tubes. These have a much wider bore (French gauge 12–14) and should only be used for aspirating the gastric contents.

3   Some tubes are made from polyvinylchloride (PVC) which tends to become brittle after prolonged contact with gastric acid. If an extended feeding period is anticipated, it would be more advisable to use a tube made from polyurethane or one of its derivatives. These are more supple and do not become brittle. Some tubes have a special coating to facilitate intubation (these need to be immersed in water rather than lubricated with jelly).

4   Introduction wires
These are provided with many of the currently available feeding tubes and are inserted in the lumen of the tube to provide additional rigidity during the intubation procedure. The 'guide' wire is withdrawn once the tube is in place and feeding is carried out in the usual way. These wires are particularly useful in patients who are difficult to intubate e.g., elderly, post-cerebrovascular accident (CVA), etc.

NB   Problems can arise when using a 'guide' wire and it is important to be aware of these (see p. 149).

5   Proximal ends
The proximal end of the tube (i.e. the end which protrudes from

the patient's nose) is either unmodified in any way or else has a Luer fitting (which may be male or female). The tube may, additionally, have an integral spigot – this is an extremely useful facility if overnight feeding or bolus feeding procedures are being used.

There is a trend to rationalise the Luer devices on all enteral feeding tubes to ensure that no confusion can exist between enteral and parenteral giving sets. This will mean that all enteral feeding tubes will, eventually, have *male* Luer ends. At present tubes with female ends are also available.

6   Distal ends

Unfortunately, these vary as much as the proximal ends! The distal end of the tube is the point at which the feeding solution enters the GI tract itself.

The end may be unmodified or there may be lateral outlets. The latter is preferable because this helps to prevent clogging and ensures a more even distribution of the feeding solution.

NB   If an introducer wire is used, great care must be taken to ensure that it does not protrude through one of the lateral outlets – this could cause a perforation of the GI tract.

Additionally, some tubes have weighted ends. These serve two purposes:

They are radio opaque and the end of the tube is readily identifiable by X-ray.

They help to maintain the tube in position. This is particularly relevant when passing a nasoduodenal tube; the weighted end helps to ensure the passage of the tube through the pylorus.

NB   *If the tube has a mercury bolus at the end this must not be incinerated* (highly toxic mercuric oxide vapour is produced). The end of the tube should be cut off and appropriate arrangements should be made for its disposal.

It is impossible to identify in this text all the feeding tubes which are currently available; local departments will have their own policies and preferences as well as holding information regarding the various products. If in doubt the personnel to contact would, normally, be:

Medical/Surgical Instrument Department
Department of Nutrition and Dietetics
Central Sterile Supplies Department (CSSD)
Nursing officer (ITU or ENT)

Giving sets

There are not so many giving sets presently available as there are feeding tubes. Great care must be taken to ensure that the entire feeding system is compatible in respect of its connections and the selection of an appropriate feeding tube may dictate the subsequent choice of a giving set. It is important to remember that bacterial contamination can occur at any of the connection points in a delivery system. These should, therefore, be kept to a minimum and handled as little as possible.

Four aspects should be considered when selecting a giving set:

1 Luer connection
Obviously this has to fit the Luer connection on the feeding tube. A male Luer connection on the tube will require a female connection on the giving set and vice-versa. Male-female Luer adaptors are available for occasional use but are *not* to be recommended for routine feeding practice.

2 Silastic insert
If an enteral feeding pump is used, a modified giving set will be required. This incorporates the use of a silastic 'insert' in the tubing which facilitates the positioning of the giving set through the rotating head of the feeding pump. Care should be taken to ensure that the insert is correctly sited in respect of the gates on the head of the pump. This will prevent the tube 'slipping' when feeding is commenced.

3 Integral reservoir
Some giving sets are marketed with an integral reservoir. This ensures that there is minimal opportunity to contaminate the feeding system because there are fewer connections.

4 Flow rate controller
This takes the form of either a screw clamp or a roller clamp. The final choice is usually a matter of individual preference. Control thus obtained is not, necessarily, highly accurate and a gate clamp may be preferred instead. It is additionally possible to regulate the flow rate mechanically:

Using an enteral feeding pump
Using an intravenous feeding pump to set the rate initially.

NB
This degree of accuracy is only required when a very slow or viscous infusion is being given.

Intravenous feeding equipment should *never* be used for enteral feeding for any reason other than to set the flow rate.

5   Burette Controller

This is a device which enables bolus feed to be delivered from a larger reservoir. The burette (which can contain varying quantities of solution) is graduated and is controlled by two clamps; the first clamp permits a measured amount of feeding solution to pass from the reservoir into the burette. The second clamp controls the rate at which the solution is administered to the patient from the burette.

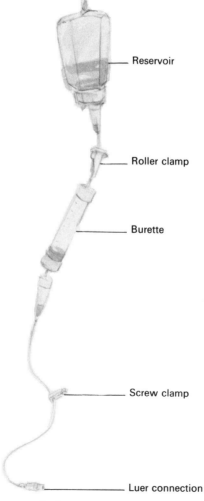

— Reservoir

— Roller clamp

— Burette

— Screw clamp

— Luer connection

Fig. 7.2   Burette-type feeding system

Reservoirs

These, too, are marketed in many different forms but there are basic requirements for reservoirs which can be considered on a general basis.

Is a reservoir necessary? Some commercial feeding companies present their products in such a way that the packaging can be used as a reservoir in its own right with minimal modification (e.g., KabiVitrum, Cow and Gate). It is generally impractical to transfer these solutions to another reservoir.

Ease of use. This is a matter of local preference. Reservoirs are manufactured in two main categories:
Bag type
Bottle type
They are both marked with volume graduations and have room to add other relevant details e.g., patient's name, hospital number and date of feed, etc.

Sterility. It is recommended that the reservoir and the giving set should be changed every 24 hours and that these should be sterile at the beginning of each feeding period. It is sometimes possible (and more economical) to re-use a feeding reservoir provided that it has been adequately sterilised. This can be done by washing the reservoir in an appropriate anionic detergent to remove all food particles. It should then be soaked in a suitable sterilising solution e.g., 10 % Milton and particular attention must be paid to the areas around the filling port and the delivery port. The most effective means of ensuring this is to fill the reservoir with sterilising solution. A bag type reservoir is more appropriate for this procedure.

NB
1 Separate giving sets should not be re-used in this way.

2 Although the reservoir and the giving set must be sterile, remember that the feeding solution is not necessarily sterile.

Size. The capacity of feeding reservoirs varies from 235 ml to 1500 ml. It is advisable to select the one which is most appropriate to local requirements taking into consideration such factors as the mobility of the patient, the ambient temperature of the ward and the amount of nursing time which is available to supervise the reservoir changeover.

Enteral feeding pumps

It is not generally necessary to use these specialised feeding pumps which are comparatively expensive and often render the patient less mobile. There are, however, instances when they are invaluable. The purpose of the pumps is to regulate the flow of the feed from the reservoir to the patient. When a pump is not used the flow rate is normally regulated by counting the drips passing through the drip chamber and adjusting the clamp on the giving set accordingly. There are two occasions when this is not satisfactory.

1 When the feeding solution has to be administered very slowly.
2 When the solution itself is very viscous and may block the feeding tube.

An enteral feeding pump is a small battery/mains operated pump with a rotating head. The only modification which is necessary in terms of the feeding equipment and solution is to ensure that the giving set has a 'silastic insert'.

The flow rate is regulated by setting the dial on the pump to the required delivery rate and then opening the clamp on the giving set. The rate is usually calibrated in terms of drops per minute. It is important to realise that different solutions may have different drop sizes and that this might affect the delivery rate.

The pump is usually taped to the patient's bedside locker or clamped to a stand. There are built-in alarm mechanisms in some models but, despite this, the delivery of the feed should be carefully checked at regular intervals.

NB It is essential constantly to ensure that the end of the feeding tube is positioned in the correct place when a pump is being used.

Practical experience has shown that pumps which have the capacity to run on battery as well as mains power are more versatile when used with most patients. It is, however, extremely important to check that the battery is adequately charged at all times. It is useful to remember that some companies will provide a temporary replacement feeding pump if any problems arise as a result of a breakdown. The manufacturers also provide clear written instructions regarding the use of individual pumps together with helpful diagrams.

Feeding solutions

It has already been emphasised on p. 143 that patients may need to be fed enterally for a variety of reasons. This means their nutritional requirements will vary accordingly and, therefore, that each patient must be assessed on an individual basis. *Average* nutritional requirements are identified in Appendix III.

It is vital to remember that these are only *average* values and, moreover, are values recorded for healthy subjects.

An enteral feeding solution is available in two different forms:

1 'Home-made' in the local diet bay, main kitchen or ward kitchen
2 Commercially prepared

The solution of choice will depend on local financial constraints, manpower resources and preparation facilities as well as upon the needs of the individual patient.

In most hospitals feeding solutions are obtained from one of the following departments:

Nutrition and Dietetics
Pharmacy
Catering

Some units hold their own supplies of feeds (or the ingredients for making up feeds) but this is not generally considered to be advisable. This is because of the need to rotate stock and avoid stock piling.

There is also the inability to take advantage of the discounts which are offered when large quantities are purchased.
NB *Outdated products must never be used.*

Home-made feeds

Each hospital or unit will have its own formula for enteral feeding which should be capable of modification to suit the needs of the individual patient. The solution should provide sources of protein, fat and carbohydrate in an acceptable total volume of fluid. The usual energy: volume ratio is 1 kcal : ml but this may vary. If long-term feeding by the enteral route is contemplated then there should also be an adequate provision of essential vitamins, minerals and trace elements. These can be added either in tablet or liquid form. If tablets are used they should be crushed very carefully to avoid any lumps which may block the tube. The solution should be shaken thoroughly before administration to make sure that there is no sediment. It is extremely difficult to produce sterile 'home-made' feeds.

Feeds can be made up from individual sources of each nutrient or from commercially prepared mixtures of nutrients. *It is very important to follow the manufacturer's instructions whichever product is used.*

Commercially prepared feeds

Many companies now market individual feeding solutions or ranges of feeding solutions which are designed for tube feeding and which are, generally, very easy to use. A comparison of the feeds which are currently available appears in Appendix V, 3.

It is very important to make sure that the manufacturer's instructions regarding the storage and administration of these solutions are carefully followed.

Administration of feeding solutions

Most hospitals have their own scheduled feeding periods and these will vary according to local policies. Once the need for enteral feeding has been established, a suitable regimen should be ordered as soon as possible. In many units it is possible to order a half day's supply of feed to avoid any delays. The feed will generally be supplied by:

Department of Nutrition and Dietetics
Pharmacy
Catering
Local ward kitchen

The feed will be sent to the ward after it has been ordered and usually enough for 24 hours will be supplied. It should be stored appropriately (e.g., a home-made feed will require refrigeration). The amount of solution presented to the patient at any one time will vary according to the individually prescribed regimen, but the following points should always be considered:

1   **Concentration.** Initially it is inadvisable to administer a feed at full strength unless it is isocaloric (i.e. provides 1 kcal: ml). In some cases even isocaloric feeds may need to be diluted with water

for the first few days. Procedures vary but the following could provide a basic guideline:

Day 1	1/4–1/2 strength
Day 2	1/2–3/4 strength
Day 3	1/2–3/4 strength
Day 4	full strength

If commercially prepared feeding solutions are used, remember to shake the can/bottle thoroughly before emptying. This will ensure that the contents are thoroughly mixed and that no sediment is left behind.

If the patient shows any sign of not tolerating the feed then the concentration should be reduced immediately.

2 **Rate of administration.** This is calculated on the basis of the total volume of solution to be administered over a 24 hour period. If bolus feeding is used then the number of individual feeding periods should be considered. In both cases this is the practice of simple arithmetic!

NB It is important to remember:
The viscosity of the feed (see p. 162)
Whether there is likely to be any time during the 24 hours when it will not be possible or practical to feed the patient (e.g., during operation, investigative X-ray procedures, etc.)
Whether an additional allowance of fluid is needed to flush the tube (bolus method only)

3 **Temperature of solution.** An ice-cold solution should not be given directly to the patient. This could cause gastric spasm with the possibility of subsequent discomfort and/or diarrhoea. The feed should be given at room temperature, but *do not overheat a solution* artificially and then cool it to the correct temperature because this could cause degradation of the nutrients.

4 **Identification of the solution.** It is extremely important that the *patient should receive the feed which has been specifically prescribed* for him. It is also vital that this should be given during a specific period of time.

In order that this can be ensured:

Labelling – the feed must be clearly identified with the patient's name, ward and the current day's date. Additional data may also be supplied but the first three items are essential and must be clearly visible.

There should also be a clear indication that the feeding system and solution is *for enteral use only*. It may help if it is labelled 'Not for intravenous use'. This, again, should be very clear and should appear where the reservoir is connected to the giving set.

Surplus feed – if any solution remains at the end of the allotted feeding period *it must be thrown away* and the rejected amount clearly recorded. This enables the next feeding period to begin on schedule thereby reducing any confusion.

5 **Modification of feeding regimen.** This can take place at any time during the feeding period and any changes should be clearly identified in the patient's notes and on any relevant feeding charts. It is important to *notify appropriate personnel of any changes to the current regimen at the earliest opportunity* to ensure continuity and minimal disruption to patient care.

NB Feeds should never be kept and given to patients for whom they are not prescribed specifically.

Monitoring

It has been stated that 'nutritional status should be considered to be an integral part of the medical management of the patient'. This means that a constant record must be kept of the patient's nutritional progress. The importance of monitoring patients on tube feeds cannot be overemphasised – sophisticated laboratory tests are meaningless if there is no accurate record of intake and output.

It is difficult to maintain suitable records without appropriate forms. These are being introduced in hospitals throughout the country and should be used whenever possible. Monitoring consists of accurate records of input and output together with information about the patient's weight, height and general clinical condition.

Input

Accuracy is the key to this exercise because this is the only way in which the medical staff can assume with certainty that the patient is receiving adequate nutrition. It is usually convenient to assess this in two ways:

1   Oral intake

Many patients who are fed enterally are still capable of eating some food orally (see p. 140). This may form an appreciable part of their nutritional intake and must, therefore, be carefully recorded. *An accurate description of the portion size eaten is vital* — if the hospital caters in 'standard portions' this can be calculated on a fractional or percentage basis. If standard portions are not used, handy measures (e.g., tablespoons) can be conveniently employed. Make sure that the measures are qualified whenever possible (e.g., heaped or level teaspoons). Do not forget to check such items as between-meal snacks (biscuits, sweets, soft drinks, etc.) as well as noting whether or not the patient takes sugar and milk on his breakfast cereal and in his tea — and, if he does, how much does he take? It is often possible to involve the patient in this exercise which, in addition to any possible therapeutic benefit, may contribute to greater accuracy.

Ideally, a specially devised chart should be kept for this purpose and a new chart should be used each day. The charts can be filed in the patient's case notes once the nutritional intakes have been assessed.

2   Tube feed intake

The main problem is to differentiate between what the patient is supposed to receive and what he actually gets. There are many occasions when the two values are different — and this is rarely the fault of the nursing staff. It is important, however, to record any such discrepancies clearly.

Again, a specially devised chart can be very helpful and this should be completed at regular intervals by the nursing staff. The prescribed nutrition can be entered in terms of individual nutrients and total volume (this will also define the strength at which the feed should be given). Any shortfall can then be recorded as a simple volume. It is then a straightforward task to analyse the nutrition which the patient has actually received.

NB   It can be easy to forget to record intakes on the relevant chart. This occurs frequently when items such as milk are taken. This would, hopefully, appear on the fluid balance chart — but may be omitted on the oral nutrition intake sheet.

Output

This is a great deal easier to record because it is a routine nursing procedure. All losses should be noted including aspirate, faeces, vomit, fistulae losses, etc. There may be requests to collect 24 hour urine samples for nitrogen analysis, etc. It is extremely important that these should be *accurately* measured, that *all* the samples should be retained during the 24 hour period and that the fluid charts should tally with the total volume of urine!

Anthropometric measurements

Nutritional requirements are calculated from the patient's height and usual body weight. In some instances the ideal body weight is used as a standard (see Appendix II). It is then possible to assess how much body weight has been lost and, more importantly, how much lean body mass has been lost. The rate of weight loss is also considered. Nutritional regimens are calculated on this basis and also take into account any increased requirements in terms of energy or specific nutrients. This can occur in cases of sepsis, severe burns, etc. (see p. 126). Certain drugs interact with various nutrients thus making the latter unavailable. This also has to be considered when calculating an appropriate regimen.

The importance of providing this information is clearly apparent. It is also necessary to weigh the patient regularly and chart any changes which may occur. This, together with the nutritional intake and output data, will provide valuable guidance about the success or failure of any individual nutritional regimen.

Problems

Unfortunately, these do occur in relation to tube feeding but are usually resolved with comparative ease. The following points are intended as a general guide rather than as an exhaustive list.

Diarrhoea

Several factors can cause diarrhoea in tube fed patients:

Concentration. The feed may be too concentrated. Try to reduce this by giving a more diluted feed.

1   Add more water to the existing amount of feed. This is only suitable if a small total volume is being given.
2   Give less feed in the same total volume and make up the difference with water.

NB The concentration of the feed may cause particular problems in patients who have had gut resections.

Antibiotic therapy. This is one of the commonest causes of diarrhoea in tube fed patients.

1   Modify the dose of antibiotic if possible.
2   Try to replace the destroyed gut flora by giving live yoghurt or blue cheese orally if this is practical.
3   Add an artificial gut flora culture to the tube feed (the Pharmacy Department will advise about this).
4   Add a suitable constipating agent to the tube feed e.g., codeine phosphate.

Bacterial contamination of the feed. Unless eggs have been used in the manufacture of the solution it is unlikely that this will be a cause of diarrhoea. The *exceptions* to this are:

1   Patients being fed via a nasoduodenal tube or stoma. This means that the gastric acid barrier has been by-passed with the possible proliferation of bacteria.

2   Patients with reduced gastric acid secretion (e.g., post-gastrectomy and those patients with achlorhydria or receiving antacid therapy such as cimetidine).

3   Patients with acute infections or sepsis and receiving broad range antibiotic therapy (see above).

4   Patients receiving immunosuppressive therapy, chemotherapy or radiation therapy.

In these cases it may be advisable to use a commercially prepared sterile feeding solution. Great care should be taken when giving the feed or otherwise handling the feeding system (see Appendix VI).

Lactose intolerance. This is unusual in most Caucasian patients, but may occur on a transient basis post-operatively. Mediterranean, Negroid and Indian races are known to have an increased intolerance to lactose. This is due to alactasia – an absence of the enzyme lactase which is needed to break down the lactose found in milk-based fluids. Diarrhoea can be avoided by giving a milk free feed which does not contain lactose. These can be locally prepared or commercially purchased (see Appendix V, 3).

Fat intolerance. Again this is unusual but can be resolved by:

1   Reducing the fat content of the feed. Increased amounts of protein and carbohydrate will need to be given in order to maintain the required energy intake.

2   Modifying the fat content of the feed by using medium chain triglycerides (MCT). This is absorbed in a different way from the long chain triglyceride (LCT) fats commonly used and may thus cure the diarrhoea.

Administration of feed. There are two ways in which this can cause diarrhoea:

1   Speed – if the feed is given too quickly, diarrhoea will ensue. Reduce the rate of administration but remember that this may affect the total volume that can be given and that the formulation may need to be adjusted accordingly.

2   Temperature – if the feed is too cold it may cause some gastric spasm with consequent intestinal hurry. Allow the feed to warm to room temperature before administration but *never* boil a solution and allow it to cool (this will cause degradation of many of the nutrients).

Maintaining the feeding tube in position

There are many patients in whom this is a recurring problem. It is, therefore, very important to remember to check at regular intervals that the tube is correctly placed.

Restless patients. Especially those who are semi-conscious, there is an automatic tendency either to withdraw the tube manually or move in such a way as to cause it to become dislodged.

1   Use a nasoduodenal tube which is longer and more difficult to remove.

2   Use the bolus or intermittent feeding method rather than continuous drip feeding.

3   Ensure that the tube is securely taped – in some cases a suture or gum adhesive may help.

Patients with unavoidable reflux.

1   Vomiting – give an appropriate anti-emetic. Attempt to ascertain whether vomiting is directly related to the administration of the feed. Review the feeding method (see p. 141).

2   Persistent cough – encourage soothing pastilles or a linctus if possible. Use a nasoduodenal tube and nurse the patient with extra pillows if this is practical.

3 Persistent hiccups — encourage the patient to suck a boiled sweet if this practical and try to distract his attention. Give a small dose of oil of peppermint and use extra pillows if this is practical.

Failure to aspirate

This can cause difficulties if the local nursing procedure dictates that the stomach contents must be checked before each feeding period commences.

The usual practice is to use a 3-way tap. The two commonest reasons for failure are:

1 **Use of a fine bore tube.** Routine aspiration technique will cause the walls of the tube to collapse with a consequent failure to obtain a sample of the gastric contents. To overcome this, use a 2 ml syringe and withdraw the contents very slowly indeed.

2 **Insecure connections.** If the feeding system is not airtight, there will be insufficient resistance to enable the gastric contents to be withdrawn. Check that the 3-way tap is securely connected and that an appropriate syringe is being used.

Blockage of tube

This can occur with comparative ease if good feeding practices are not followed. Some common causes are:

'Lumpy' solution. *All* feeds should be thoroughly shaken/blended to ensure a smooth consistency.

Unmodified distal end of tube in contact with gastric acid. The protein in the feed becomes denatured when it is in contact with gastric acid (the beginning of the digestion process). If the tube only has one terminal outlet, it can become blocked in this way.

Viscous feed being administered without a pump. If the feed is very thick it will tend to flow rather slowly and can cause a gradual blockage of the tube. This can be a particular problem if a fine bore tube is used.

Residue not cleared from tube after bolus feeding. When this method of feeding is used the tube should always be flushed with a small amount of water (25 − 50 ml) before and after feeding.

In all the instances mentioned above the following steps should be taken to solve the problem.

1   Flush the tube through with water. This will clear most blockages provided it is done promptly.

2   Check the position of the end of the tube – change it if necessary.

3   Check that an appropriate tube is being used (see p. 146). Change it if necessary and practical.

4   Consider using an enteral feeding pump if the solution is very thick.

Care of the patient

Many problems confront the patient who is being tube fed. Some of these have been discussed on p. 161. It is important to remember that tube feeding is not a natural way of receiving nutrition and, quite often, patients do not realise that they are, in fact, being fed. Close attention should be paid to the following points:

1   **Explanation.** This is essential and must be repeated as often as is necessary. In particular the intubation procedure should be explained very carefully because it can be a distressing experience for both nurse and patient if complete co-operation is not obtained.

Bowel function is frequently altered when a patient receives tube feeding. Again, this should be carefully explained so that he knows what to expect – and that there is no need to worry about any apparent abnormality. It is vital that the patient should realise the importance of the feeding process and that he should receive constant reassurance and encouragement.

2   **Meal times.** Some patients may find it upsetting to watch others eating normal meals when they are unable to do so. It may be possible to move an individual patient. Alternatively, some distraction may be provided at meal times (the Voluntary Services Department or the League of Friends may be able to help).

3   **Awareness of the tube itself.** If a tube is positioned and taped in such a way as to be constantly uncomfortable or in the patient's line of vision, it is likely to cause resentment. The tube could be taped up the bridge of the nose and secured to the

forehead with a small clear tape dressing. It may be worth considering whether there is any need for a large, occlusive dressing.

4 **Mouth care.** Patients frequently complain of an unpleasant mouth and close attention should be paid to this. Refreshing mouth washes should be given whenever practical. Particular care should be given to dental hygiene.

Conclusion

Tube feeding is a realistic and practicable means of feeding patients who are unable to achieve their required daily nutritional intake by the oral route. It is a method of feeding which involves the use of specific equipment and feeding solutions which have been carefully designed for the purpose. There is also the need for accurate monitoring of the patient's progress. Despite this, it is not difficult and is to be preferred to intravenous feeding whenever possible. This is because it is not associated with the same infection complications and is, physiologically, a more acceptable way of providing nutrition to a compromised patient.

8
Parenteral or Intravenous Feeding

Introduction

Parenteral or intravenous feeding is required to meet a patient's nutritional needs when adequate food cannot be instilled into or absorbed from the gastrointestinal tract. About 5 % of all hospital admissions may require such management and indeed it can be life-saving. It is, however, potentially more hazardous than enteral feeding and its successful use requires great expertise. The clinical conditions where its use is indicated are given in Table 8.1. In grossly wasted patients, intravenous feeding may last for many weeks. Initial weight gain in the first days is usually due to rehydration; after this a gain of 1 kilogram per week is good progress, as the process of rebuilding lost body tissue is slow. A successful outcome is dependent upon good vascular access and prevention of both catheter-related sepsis and electrolyte imbalances.

Clinical conditions which may specifically exclude its use are:

Cardiac failure
Severe liver damage
Shock
Severe blood disorders
Uncontrolled diabetes mellitus
Malaria

Vascular access

The solutions used for parenteral nutrition are concentrated and will sclerose small arm or leg veins. They must be infused into the patient via a major vein. Poor morale and loss of confidence are common in those patients who have become undernourished. A clear explanation of the therapy, stressing the beneficial effects on physical strength and general well-being and the comfort of the intravenous catheter, once inserted, will allay many fears.

During feeding the prevention of infection is vital as not only will the nutrient solutions readily support bacterial growth but, in addition, catheter insertion sites must be meticulously dressed to avoid infections. By attention to detail the nurse can help prevent many of these complications.

Table 8.1   Clinical situations in which parenteral nutrition may
be beneficial

Bowel diseases	Intestinal fistula
	Short bowel syndrome
	Inflammatory bowel disease
	Loss of motility
Pancreatic disease	Acute pancreatitis
	Pancreatic abscess
	Pancreatic pseudocyst or fistula
Trauma	Major burns
	Multiple trauma
Surgery	Restoration of weight loss before surgery, following major surgery or complications in the post-operative period.
	Failure to achieve the required nutrient intake within five post-operative days.

Nutrient solutions

There are many available solutions to provide the various
components required for parenteral nutrition. The composition of
a feeding regimen will vary according to each patient's special
needs.

Energy sources.   The principal two are glucose and fat solutions.
Glucose is the main energy source and its effect must be carefully
monitored as a high blood sugar is not desirable. The solutions
available are given in Appendix VII, 2. Most have *some* electrolytes
added. The fat solutions are of 10% and 20% and fat soluble
vitamins should be added to these solutions.

Nitrogen/protein sources.   The commonly used commercial
solutions are given in Appendix VII, 2. The nitrogen and electrolyte
content also varies and must be considered when planning a regimen.
    The energy and nitrogen requirements are closely linked. The
nitrogen loss is assessed from all sources and calculated in grams.
Requirements exceed this figure by 3–5 g of nitrogen and the
energy requirements are then calculated according to the clinical
state of the patient.

Vitamin supplements.   The recommended daily needs and the
contents of available solutions are noted (Appendix VII, 3). Folate

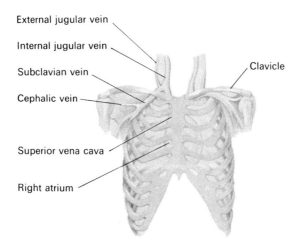

External jugular vein

Internal jugular vein

Subclavian vein

Cephalic vein

Clavicle

Superior vena cava

Right atrium

Fig. 8.1 For central venous feeding the catheter tip will lie at the lower end of the superior vena cava, where rapid dilution with blood reduces the damaging effects of the irritant nutrient solutions.

The most common site of catheter insertion is the subclavian vein although the jugular veins and the cephalic vein are sometimes used. The veins of the arm are avoided as friction from the catheter during arm movements may damage the veins.

and Vitamin B_{12} supplements are always needed in addition to the commercial solution of choice. Some vitamins are easily degraded by exposure to light, therefore feeding solutions should be covered appropriately.

Complications

The complications are potentially many, varied and perhaps lethal, yet avoidable with proper understanding and good technique. (See Table 8.2.)

Infection

Infection is such a serious and constant threat that all those involved in the administration of parenteral nutrition need to be vigilant to prevent *any* microbial contamination. Organisms may gain access to the circulation either through the lumen of the catheter, from the fluids or connections in the administration set, or around the catheter entry site. Protocols for management should be effective but simple enough to be performed in any situation, whether the intensive care unit, the general ward or the patient's home.

Infusion fluids

Stability problems and varying individual needs preclude the commercial production, on a general scale, of single containers of all nutrients. Therefore, the nurse may be required to change up to eight containers a day having first made additions of vitamins and trace elements. Even careful handwashing and the use of sterile gloves are insufficient to prevent contamination by skin cells and hair when such additions are made on the ward. Furthermore, the need to infuse a nitrogen source concurrently with a source of non-nitrogen calories results in infusions which are difficult to control and subject to mechanical problems, such as catheter blockage, requiring extra manipulation of the infusion system. It is the pharmacist's responsibility to dispense nutrients in the most suitable form for administration and the development of the single, collapsible, non-vented, three litre container in which all the patient's daily nutritional requirements are mixed together by the pharmacist within the bacteriologically-controlled environment of a laminar air flow cabinet, is a major advance. Sometimes it is possible to add fat emulsion to these bags, however such emulsions are unstable in the presence of elevated amounts of calcium and magnesium and usually require separate infusion.

Infusion system

Many types of administration sets and associated equipment are available although not all are suitable for parenteral nutrition. The system should incorporate minimal connections, and those which are essential should be Luer locking. Multiple tap systems are both dangerous and unnecessary, as one-piece administration sets with two or three limbs for simultaneous infusions are available.

Microbe retentive filters with a membrane pore size of 0.1 or 0.2 micron have been advocated as valuable aids to infection control. However, these provide no protection against the entry of organisms through the connection below the filter and around the catheter. Furthermore, fat emulsions cannot be infused through them.

During the daily changing of the administration set it is advisable to handle the connections with sterile gloves, following disinfection with a suitable agent such as Chlorhexidine 0.5 % in 70 % spirit.

Care of catheter insertion site

The intravenous catheter forms a direct link between the external environment and the venous circulation and the entry site requires scrupulous care. The dressing covering the site should be changed three times weekly unless the catheter has been tunnelled, in which case a weekly change is sufficient. After observing the entry site for redness, discharge or other signs of local infection, and checking the security of the sutures anchoring the catheter, skin debris should be removed with an agent such as acetone or chlorhexidine 0.5 % in 70 % spirit using non-touch technique. Povidone iodine, applied to the skin around the entry site, provides effective anti-bacterial, anti-fungal protection. The dry powder from an aerosol spray is the most convenient form.

Any infection associated with parenteral nutrition demands a close examination of current procedures, preferably in conjunction with a bacteriologist or infection control nurse.

Catheter insertion into the subclavian, jugular or cephalic vein (see diagram p. 167) requires the patient to lie flat with no pillow, possibly with a rolled towel placed longitudinally down the back causing the shoulders to fall back. In addition the foot of the bed should be elevated, to increase venous filling and reduce the risk of air embolism. Understandably, this position is most uncomfortable, especially for those patients with surgical wounds. Adequate analgesia, possibly combined with mild sedation, not only relieves the discomfort but permits the patient to lie still so reducing the risk of damage to adjacent structures as the doctor is locating the vein.

The catheter is made of silicone rubber because it may have to remain in place for months. Its placement requires great expertise, the procedure being done in the Operating Theatre under strict asepsis to prevent infection being introduced. The position of the catheter tip is checked by X-ray to ensure it is in the correct position before nutrient solutions are infused. The part of the catheter remaining is then tunnelled under the skin as this reduces infective complications later. The entry site is kept clean. With this technique the patient still has free movement of his arms and shoulders and the entry site is on a flat convenient surface on the anterior chest wall.

Technical complications

Although complications of catheter insertion may occur initially, the incidence reduces to almost nil with experience and emphasises the importance of a chest X-ray to detect any possible technical complications before feeding commences. Problems may occur during insertion of the catheter or whilst parenteral nutrition is in progress. Accidental arterial puncture, air embolism, a pneumothorax or damage to the brachial plexus may occur. Further the catheter tip may be misplaced within the venous circulation, or outside into the mediastinum or pleura.

The incidence of catheter infection also varies with experience, but may occur in up to one-quarter of all patients. Tunnelling of the catheter and excellent nursing care of the entry site greatly reduce the incidence. When infection is present it may be at a site other than the catheter, such as an intra-abdominal abscess or a urinary tract or chest infection, and all possible causes must be excluded or treated as appropriate. Bacteriological swabs should be taken from all exposed sites – particularly where the catheter enters the skin. If no cause is found then the feeding line should be removed. Usually within two days the fever settles and antibiotics are not used. The catheter tip is sent for bacteriological culture, and generally *Staphylococcus aureus* or *Candida albicans* are the infective organisms isolated. A new catheter is then inserted through a new entry site.

Metabolic complications

Metabolic complications are potentially many. A raised blood sugar – hyperglycaemia – may lead to eventual dehydration and coma. Regular monitoring of blood and urine sugar will prevent

Table 8.2   Complications of parenteral feeding

Catheter insertion	Anterior puncture
	Nerve injury to brachial plexus or phrenic nerve
	Pneumothorax
	Haemothorax
	Hydrothorax – infusion of solution into the chest
	Air embolism
	Haematoma at the site of insertion
Catheter Sepsis	
Metabolic	Dehydration
	Raised blood sugar
	Raised serum potassium
	Deficiencies of electrolytes, vitamins and folate
Transient changes in liver function	

this, while a rising blood sugar may be controlled by reducing the rate of infusion or in some cases with insulin.

Detailed records must be kept to show:

1 Amount of nitrogen, electrolytes, energy, water, vitamins, essential fats and trace elements infused.

2 Output of nitrogen, sodium, potassium, urea and fluid from all sources.

Catheter patency and infusion

The potential dangers of rapid infusion are increased by the use of three litre containers because of the large volume of hypertonic fluid which could pass into the patient. Suddenly slowing or stopping the infusion is equally dangerous and may cause a reactive hypoglycaemia especially if the patient is receiving insulin. Accurate flow control is therefore critical and it is the nurse's responsibility to select the most appropriate means of doing this.

The safest and most effective method of controlling the infusion is by a volumetric infusion pump. Whilst these are expensive and require special administration sets, problems associated with other devices are avoided. For example, drop counting controllers are often inaccurate as no account is taken of drop size which varies according to fluid viscosity. Peristaltic pumps often have a high pressure output and may rupture the catheter or cause disconnections if the catheter blocks or becomes kinked. Less expensive, disposable regulators are effective but require recalibration for hypertonic solutions. Measured volume administration sets are useful but require frequent checking and must have a 'shut off' valve at the fluid chamber outlet to prevent air entering the tubing should the fluid run out. The most inaccurate, unsafe and frustrating method of controlling the infusion is by the plastic roller valve on the administration set and it is most unwise to depend on these to control such potentially hazardous therapy.

Catheter blockage will occur if the infusion flow is stopped by an empty collapsible container, closed flow control valve, the catheter twisting inside a hub or reflux of blood into the catheter. The latter commonly occurs during gravity infusions when ambulant patients lower the infusion stand to pass through doors resulting in the drip chamber being too low to maintain a satisfactory head of pressure.

Patients may be encouraged to exercise more freely if parenteral nutrition is discontinued for several hours during the day. To maintain patency the catheter is filled with a solution of heparinised saline (Hepsal) and closed by a Luer locking cap. Complications may occur if blood is drawn back into the catheter during this procedure when the clamp is applied to change from the empty syringe to the catheter cap. Injecting the drug directly through a latex-covered Luer locking spigot with a fine 25G needle avoids this problem.

Even during well managed infusions catheter blockage remains an occasional complication. Flushing the catheter with normal saline from a 2 ml syringe may be helpful. Silicone rubber catheters require special care, with a very gradual increase in pressure to avoid splitting the soft material. Should these measures fail, flushing with Hepsal may be of value; failing this Urokinase 5000 units diluted in 3 ml normal saline instilled into the catheter for 30 minutes, before being aspirated, is often successful. This is a medical procedure and should be undertaken only by those experienced in the use of central venous catheters.

Infusion pumps which include alarms for occlusion, in-line air and empty containers assist in preventing some of these complications, however they do not replace observation by the skilled nurse.

Home parenteral nutrition

For a small number of patients who require parenteral nutrition for many months or years, it is usual for therapy to continue at home. Usually these people have lost the ability to remain healthy by absorbing nutrients through the gastrointestinal tract either because of extensive resection or disease or because of abnormalities in gut motility. Such treatment requires considerable organisation and the nurse plays a major role in training the patient, selecting safe equipment and establishing liaison with health care professionals in the community. Whilst all these functions are important, perhaps the most critical nursing responsibility lies in helping the patient and his family make the emotional adjustment to a new way of living. To do this she must be aware of relationships within the family and understand their attitude towards parenteral nutrition. A warm, caring atmosphere in which views can be openly expressed and respected can only be created when the nurse feels confident in her own abilities and receives good support from members of other disciplines involved in the patient's care.

Remember when feeding patients parenterally:

Maintain an even rate of administration to prevent swings in the blood sugar levels. Never 'catch up'.

Do not suddenly discontinue the infusion unless an alternative source of dextrose can be provided, i.e. sweet drinks (if allowed) or dextrose 10 % by central or peripheral vein.

Patients who receive overnight infusions only must have the flow rate tapered (50 ml per hour for the last 30 – 60 minutes or give them breakfast if they can eat it) as prescribed, before discontinuing the infusion.

Observe temperature, pulse and respiratory rate every four hours.

Test the urine for sugar and ketones every 6 hours.

Weigh patient daily.

Record fluid balance accurately.

Change giving set daily.

Change insertion site dressing weekly or more frequently if it becomes wet or loose.

Do not give blood or drugs or attempt to measure central venous pressure through the catheter.

All staff handling the catheter, infusion system or fluid container must use aseptic technique.

Change the short extension tube weekly.

Peripheral venous feeding

Summary of indications

Short-term therapy 10 – 14 days. Patients with limited nutritional requirements, up to 2000 cal and 9 g nitrogen daily, and at least four good peripheral veins.

Sometimes patients who are fairly well nourished require a short period of intravenous feeding to provide support whilst the bowel is rested and cannot be used. If these patients have good peripheral veins, it may be possible to avoid the need for a central venous catheter by infusing nutrients into the peripheral circulation. Some patients may receive nutrients in this manner until it is convenient to insert a central venous catheter for long-term use.

Amino acid and concentrated dextrose solutions are hypertonic and damage the veins. To avoid this damage amino acids are infused simultaneously with the fat emulsion Intralipid (10 % or 20 %), which is isotonic with plasma and has a neutral pH, and dextrose 10% is infused simultaneously with normal saline. Up to 80% of daily calorie requirements can be provided as Intralipid. Even with these precautions, painful thrombophlebitis may develop and become septic, and strict attention must be paid to protocol. In addition to the aseptic procedures for changing containers and giving sets, special care is required in the technique of cannula insertion and maintenance. A cannula will be inserted into each arm. Attached to each of these will be a short extension tube capped by a Luer locking spigot. The infusion will rotate 24 hourly between the two sites, patency in the non-operative cannula being maintained by an injection of Hepsal 2 ml. No more than two infusions must be given into each vein and when removed the cannula tip should be cultured.

Appendix I

Summary of general guidelines for good nutrition

1 Achieve ideal body weight for height by modifying overall calorie intake

2 Reduce intakes of the following:
   Refined carbohydrates, e.g., sugar, sweets, etc.
   Fats
   a Visible, e.g., butter, oil, fat or meat, etc.
   b Invisible, e.g., cakes, pastries, full fat milk, etc.
   Salt
   a At table
   b High salt containing foods, e.g., cheese, ham, etc.
   Alcohol

3 Increase intakes of the following:
   Unrefined carbohydrate
   a Pulses, e.g., peas, dried beans, lentils
   b Fruits and other vegetables including potatoes
   c Cereals, e.g., flour, rice
   d Nuts
   Fish and chicken

4 Take adequate exercise

Appendix II

DESIRABLE WEIGHTS OF ADULTS according to height and frame

Height without shoes			Desirable weight in kilograms and pounds (in indoor clothing). ages 25 and over					
			Small frame		Medium frame		Large frame	
metres	ft	in	kg	lb	kg	lb	kg	lb
Men								
1.550	5	1	50.8—54.4	112—120	53.5—58.5	118—129	57.2—64	126—141
1.575	5	2	52.2—55.8	115—123	54.9—60.3	121—133	58.5—65.3	129—144
1.600	5	3	53.5—57.2	118—126	56.2—61.7	124—136	59.9—67.1	132—148
1.625	5	4	54.9—58.5	121—129	57.6—63	127—139	61.2—68.9	135—152
1.650	5	5	56.2—60.3	124—133	59—64.9	130—143	62.6—70.8	138—156
1.675	5	6	58.1—62.1	128—137	60.8—66.7	134—147	64.4—73	142—161
1.700	5	7	59.9—64	132—141	62.6—68.9	138—152	66.7—75.3	147—166
1.725	5	8	61.7—65.8	136—145	64.4—70.8	142—156	68.5—77.1	151—170
1.750	5	9	63.5—68	140—150	66.2—72.6	146—160	70.3—78.9	155—174
1.775	5	10	65.3—69.9	144—154	68—74.8	150—165	72.1—81.2	159—179
1.800	5	11	67.1—71.7	148—158	69.9—77.1	154—170	74.4—83.5	164—184
1.825	6	0	68.9—73.5	152—162	71.7—79.4	158—175	76.2—85.7	168—189
1.850	6	1	70.8—75.7	156—167	73.5—81.6	162—180	78.5—88	173—194
1.875	6	2	72.6—77.6	160—171	75.7—83.5	167—185	80.7—90.3	178—199
1.900	6	3	74.4—79.4	164—175	78.1—86.2	172—190	82.7—92.5	182—204
Women								
1.425	4	8	41.7—44.5	92—98	43.5—48.5	96—107	47.2—54	104—119
1.450	4	9	42.6—45.8	94—101	44.5—49.9	98—110	48.1—55.3	106—122
1.475	4	10	43.5—47.2	96—104	45.8—51.3	101—113	49.4—56.7	109—125
1.500	4	11	44.9—48.5	99—107	47.2—52.6	104—116	50.8—58.1	112—128
1.525	5	0	46.3—49.9	102—110	48.5—54	107—119	52.2—59.4	115—131
1.550	5	1	47.6—51.3	105—113	49.9—55.3	110—122	53.5—60.8	118—134
1.575	5	2	49—52.6	108—116	51.3—57.2	113—126	54.9—62.6	121—138
1.600	5	3	50.3—54	111—119	52.6—59	116—130	56.7—64.4	125—142
1.625	5	4	51.7—55.8	114—123	54.4—61.2	120—135	58.5—66.2	129—146
1.650	5	5	53.5—57.6	118—127	56.2—63	124—139	60.3—68	133—150
1.675	5	6	55.3—59.4	122—131	58.1—64.9	128—143	62.1—69.9	137—154
1.700	5	7	57.2—61.2	126—135	59.9—66.7	132—147	64—71.7	141—158
1.725	5	8	59—63.5	130—140	61.7—68.5	136—151	65.8—73.9	145—163
1.750	5	9	60.8—65.3	134—144	63.5—70.3	140—155	67.6—76.2	149—168
1.775	5	10	62.6—67.1	138—148	65.3—72.1	144—159	69.4—79	153—174

Based on weights of insured persons in the United States associated with lowest mortality (*Statist bull Metrop Life Insur Co.* 40, Nov–Dec. 1959).

Appendix III

Recommended daily amounts of food energy and some nutrients for population groups in the United Kingdom

Age range [a] years	Occupational category	Energy [b] MJ	Energy [b] Kcal	Protein [c] g	Thiamin mg	Riboflavin mg	Nicotinic acid equivalents mg [d]	Total folate [e] µg	Ascorbic acid mg	Vitamin A retinol equivalents µg [f]	Vitamin D [g] cholecalciferol µg	Calcium mg	Iron mg
Boys													
under 1					0.3	0.4	5	50	20	450	7.5	600	6
1		5.0	1200	30	0.5	0.6	7	100	20	300	10	600	7
2		5.75	1400	35	0.6	0.7	8	100	20	300	10	600	7
3–4		6.5	1560	39	0.6	0.8	9	100	20	300	10	600	8
5–6		7.25	1740	43	0.7	0.9	10	200	20	300	(g)	600	10
7–8		8.25	1980	49	0.8	1.0	11	200	20	400	(g)	600	10
9–11		9.5	2280	57	0.9	1.2	14	200	25	575	(g)	700	12
12–14		11.0	2640	66	1.1	1.4	16	300	25	725	(g)	700	12
15–17		12.0	2880	72	1.2	1.7	19	300	30	750	(g)	600	12
Girls													
under 1					0.3	0.4	5	50	20	450	7.5	600	6
1		4.5	1100	27	0.4	0.6	7	100	20	300	10	600	7
2		5.5	1300	32	0.5	0.7	8	100	20	300	10	600	7
3–4		6.25	1500	37	0.6	0.8	9	100	20	300	10	600	8
5–6		7.0	1680	42	0.7	0.9	10	200	20	300	(g)	600	10
7–8		8.0	1900	47	0.8	1.0	11	200	20	400	(g)	600	10
9–11		8.5	2050	51	0.8	1.2	14	300	25	575	(g)	700	12 (i)
12–14		9.0	2150	53	0.9	1.4	16	300	25	725	(g)	700	12 (i)
15–17		9.0	2150	53	0.9	1.7	19	300	30	750	(g)	600	12 (i)

Men												
18–34	Sedentary	10.5	2510	63	1.0	1.6	18	300	30	750	(g)	500	10
	Moderately active	12.0	2900	72	1.2	1.6	18	300	30	750	(g)	500	10
	Very active	14.0	3350	84	1.3	1.6	18	300	30	750	(g)	500	10
35–64	Sedentary	10.0	2400	60	1.0	1.6	18	300	30	750	(g)	500	10
	Moderately active	11.5	2750	69	1.1	1.6	18	300	30	750	(g)	500	10
	Very active	14.0	3350	84	1.3	1.6	18	300	30	750	(g)	500	10
65–74	Assuming a	10.0	2400	60	1.0	1.6	18	300	30	750	(g)	500	10
75+	sedentary life	9.0	2150	54	0.9	1.6	18	300	30	750	(g)	500	10
Women												
18–54	Most occupations	9.0	2150	54	0.9	1.3	15	300	30	750	(g)	500	12(i)
	Very active	10.5	2500	62	1.0	1.3	15	300	30	750	(g)	500	12(i)
55–74	Assuming a	8.0	1900	47	0.8	1.3	15	300	30	750	(g)	500	10
75+	sedentary life	7.0	1680	42	0.7	1.3	15	300	30	750	(g)	500	10
	Pregnancy	10.0	2400	60	1.0	1.6	18	500	60	750	10	1200(h)	13
	Lactation	11.5	2750	69	1.1	1.8	21	400	60	1200	10	1200	15

Notes

(a) Since the recommendations are average amounts, the figures for each age range represent the amounts recommended at the middle of the range. Within each age range, younger children will need less, and older children more, than the amount recommended.

(b) Megajoules (10⁴ joules). Calculated from the relation 1 kilocalorie = 4.184 kilojoules, that is to say, 1 megajoule = 240 kilocalories.

(c) Recommended amounts have been calculated as 10% of the recommendations for energy.

(d) 1 nicotinic acid equivalent = 1 mg available nicotinic acid or 60 mg tryptophan.

(e) No information is available about requirements of children for folate. Graded amounts are recommended between the figure shown for infants under 1 year, which is based upon the average folate content of mature human milk, and the 300 μg daily which is suggested for adults.

(f) 1 retinol equivalent = 1 μg retinol or 6 μgβ carotene or 12 μg other biologically active carotenoids.

(g) No dietary sources may be necessary for children and adults who are sufficiently exposed to sunlight, but during the winter children and adolescents should receive 10 μg (400 i.u.) daily by supplementation. Adults with inadequate exposure to sunlight, for example those who are housebound, may also need a supplement of 10 μg daily.

(h) For the third trimester only.

(i) This intake may not be sufficient for 10% of girls and women with large menstrual losses.

Appendix IV

Increase in energy expenditure following injury
and illness

Elective Surgery	24%
Skeletal Trauma	32%
Blunt Trauma	37%
Trauma with Steroids	61%
Sepsis	79%
Burns	< 131%

NB Each $1°$ rise in temperature increases energy expenditure by 10%.

Appendix V

1 High protein, high calorie supplements

Fortified fruit juice

150 ml   fruit juice ⎫
50 g   Caloreen* ⎬ = 1 portion
50 g   sugar   ⎭

Content per portion ≃ 450 calories

Fortified soup

100 ml   strained soup ⎫
25 g   skimmed   milk │
         powder   ⎬ = 1 portion
25 g   Caloreen*   │
1   egg   ⎭

Content per portion ≃ 320 calories
                     16 g protein

Fortified milk pudding

150 ml   milk   ⎫
50 ml   double cream   │
25 g   Caloreen*   ⎬ = 1 portion
25 g   sugar   │
15 g   ground rice or semolina, etc. ⎭

NB Do not boil. More milk can be added if this is to be
taken through a straw.

Content per portion ≃ 575 calories
                     7.5 g protein

Fortified egg flip

150 ml   milk   ⎫
1   egg   │
25 g   skimmed milk powder ⎬ = 1 portion
50 ml   double cream   ⎭

NB Brandy can be added if wished (subject to
medical approval).
Sugar can also be added.

Content per portion ≃ 485 calories
                     21 g protein

*Any similar product can be used in place of Caloreen
e.g., Maxijul, Calonutrin, etc.

2 Commercial supplementary feeding formulae

Nutritional composition per 100 ml

Manufacturer	Product	Package size	Energy (kcal)	Nitrogen (g)	Protein (g)	Fat (g)	CHO (g)	Na^+ (mmol)	K^+ (mmol)
Carnation Foods	Build-Up	37.5 g	107	0.96	6.06	3.77	13.09	3.93	7.02
Cow and Gate	Fortimel*	200 ml	100	1.50	9.70	2.10	10.40	2.20	5.10
	Fortisip-Energy Plus*	200 ml	150	0.78	5.00	6.50	17.90	3.50	3.80
	Fortisip-Standard*	200 ml	100	0.63	4.00	4.00	12.00	3.50	3.80
Farley Health Products	Flavoured Complan*†**	454 g	191	0.95	5.94	5.71	12.98	6.71	9.93
	Unflavoured Complan*	454 g	190	0.93	5.81	5.48	13.33	6.52	10.00
KabiVitrum	Nutrauxil*	200 ml	100	0.61	3.80	3.40	13.80	3.30	3.20
MCP Pharmaceuticals	Salvimulsin MCT*	500 ml	100	0.76	4.80	3.00	13.50	4.00	3.00
Oxford Nutrition	Vitadrink*	250 ml	92	0.62	3.88	2.90	12.00	2.16	3.80
Wyeth Laboratories	Frutein†*	200 ml	65	0.48	3.00	–	14.00	2.06	2.06

Nutritional composition per 100 g

Manufacturer	Product	Package size	Energy (kcal)	Nitrogen (g)	Protein (g)	Fat (g)	CHO (g)	Na⁺ (mmol)	K⁺ (mmol)
Cow and Gate	Comminuted Chicken	110 g	60	1.20	7.50	3.00	—	0.40	1.30
Glaxo	Casilan	250 g	376	14.40	90.00	1.80	0.50	TR	TR
Scientific Hospital Supplies	Maxamaid Complete	200 g	350	4.80	30.00	—	65.00	25.20	21.53
	Maxipro HBV	1 kg	360	14.10	88.00	4.00	TR	10.00	11.50
Unigreg	Forceval Protein	15 g	366	8.60	55.00	0.90	30.00	5.20	1.28
Abbott Laboratories	Polycose—Liquid†† *	59 g	200	—	—	—	50.00	3.04	—
	–Powder	350 g	380	—	—	—	94.00	4.78	—
Beecham Products	Hycal†† *	170 ml	250	—	—	—	113.60	0.60	0.016
Cow and Gate	Fortical†† *	200 ml	246	—	—	—	61.50	0.30	0.20
	Polycal**	400 g	380	—	—	—	94.50	2.17	1.28
Geistlich	Calonutrin	100 g	410	—	—	—	100.00	4.00	0.30
Roussel	Caloreen	100 g	400	—	—	—	100.00	1.80	0.30
Scientific Hospital Supplies	Duocal	100 g	470	—	—	22.3	72.70	1.22	0.08
	Maxijul (*–**)	100 g	375	—	—	—	96.00	2.00	0.10

Nutritional composition per 100 ml

Cow and Gate	MCT Oil	1000 ml	830	—	98.00	—	—	—
Duncan Flockhart	Prosparol	1000 ml	450	—	50.00	—	0.7	—
Mead Johnson	MCT Oil	950 ml	830	—	98.00	—	—	—
Scientific Hospital Supplies	Calogen	2000 ml	450	—	50.00	—	0.9	0.5
	Liquigen	2000 ml	400	—	52.00	—	1.5	0.7

Domestic nutritional supplements: composition per 100 g

Milk—fresh, whole ††		65	0.52	3.30	3.80	4.70	2.17	3.84
— dried, powder		490	4.12	26.30	26.30	39.40	19.13	32.50
— skimmed, dried powder		355	5.70	36.40	1.30	52.80	23.90	71.73
Double cream ††		447	0.23	1.50	48.20	2.00	1.17	2.02
Egg – standard raw	50 g	73	0.96	6.15	5.45	TR	3.04	1.79
Cooking oil ††		899	—	—	99.90	—	TR	TR
Sugar		394	—	—	—	105.00	TR	TR

* Ready to use formulations
† Average figure
NB. Some manufacturers recommend that certain tube feeding • Formulae reconstituted according to manufacturer's instructions
formulae can be used for sip feeding regimens, †† Composition per 100 ml
** Alternative packaging available

This table is only intended as a guide to some of the nutritional products which are currently available. Further information regarding their use should be obtained from the dietitian.

3 Tube feeding formulae (for enteral use only): nutritional composition per package

Manufacturer	Product	State (3)	Package size	Dilution (1)	Packages per litre	Energy (kcal)	N (g)	Pro (g)	CHO (g)	Fat (g)	Na (mmol)	K (mmol)	Ca (mmol)	P (mmol)	Mg (mmol)	Fe (mmol)	Zn (mmol)	Cl (mmol)
Abbott Labs	Enrich*†	L	237 ml	—	4.2	260	1.51	9.4	38.3	8.8	8.69	9.48	4.25	5.44	2.78	0.05	0.06	9.52
	Ensure – Standard*(2)	L	237 ml	—	4.2	250	1.40	8.8	34.3	8.8	8.69	9.48	3.25	4.16	2.05	0.04	0.06	9.52
	– Plus*	L	237 ml	—	4.2	355	2.08	13.0	47.3	12.6	11.70	14.10	3.75	4.80	3.07	0.06	0.08	13.16
	Osmolite**(2)	L	237 ml	—	4.2	250	1.40	8.8	34.3	9.1	5.65	6.15	3.25	4.16	2.05	0.03	0.05	5.60
	Two CAL HN*	L	237 ml	—	4.2	475	3.16	19.8	51.4	21.5	10.86	14.10	6.25	8.00	4.10	0.08	0.08	10.36
Bristol-Myers	Isocal*	L	250 ml	—	4.0	252	1.28	8.0	31.5	10.5	5.45	8.01	3.74	4.03	2.06	0.04	0.04	7.02
Cow and Gate	Fortison																	
	– Standard	L	500 ml	—	2.0	500	3.15	20.0	60.0	20.0	17.39	19.23	6.25	8.00	3.12	0.09	0.05	11.25
	– Energy Plus	L	500 ml	—	2.0	750	3.90	25.0	89.5	32.5	17.39	19.23	6.25	8.00	3.12	0.09	0.05	11.25
	– Low Sodium	L	500 ml	—	2.0	500	3.15	20.0	60.0	20.0	5.43	19.23	6.25	8.00	3.12	0.09	0.05	3.50
	– Soya*	L	500 ml	—	2.0	500	3.15	20.0	60.0	20.0	17.39	19.23	6.25	8.00	3.12	0.09	0.05	11.25
	Pre-Fortison	L	500 ml	—	2.0	250	1.55	10.0	30.0	10.0	8.69	9.61	3.12	4.16	3.12	0.09	0.05	5.64
KabiVitrum	Nutrauxil	L	500 ml	—	2.0	500	3.04	19.0	69.0	17.0	16.50	16.00	6.50	10.00	2.50	0.09	0.05	16.50
MCP Pharm.	Salvimulsin MCT*	L	500 ml	—	2.0	500	3.84	24.0	67.5	15.0	20.00	15.00	5.00	7.00	3.00	0.05	0.04	14.00
Merck	Triosorbon*	P	85 g	+400 ml	2.5	400	2.59	16.1	47.6	16.1	17.00	17.00	5.10	7.65	2.98	0.06	0.04	21.25
Oxford Nut.	Hipernutril MCT*	P	90 g	+500 ml	2.0	400	3.67	22.9	49.7	12.5	17.80	17.80	2.10	5.70	1.40	0.03	0.04	17.00
	Stressnutril	P	91 g	+450 ml	2.2	416	2.50	16.0	50.5	14.5	18.00	13.00	5.00	8.50	3.00	0.03	0.03	8.00

Manufacturer	Product	State	Quantity	Dilution														
Roussel	– Iso	L	375 ml	—	2.6	375	1.68	10.5	49.0	15.4	5.70	14.40	5.62	5.05	1.84	0.05	0.05	11.03
	– 400*	L	375 ml	+125 ml	2.0	400	2.40	15.0	55.0	13.4	10.50	12.38	5.00	7.36	2.01	0.03	0.04	7.00
	– Favour*	L	375 ml	+125 ml	2.0	375	2.25	14.1	52.5	12.4	11.40	10.60	4.40	4.80	3.07	0.05	0.04	12.06
	– Protein Rich	L	375 ml	+125 ml	2.0	500	4.80	30.0	70.0	11.0	12.75	21.55	3.25	8.96	1.84	0.07	0.05	13.16
Scientific Hospital Supplies	Enteral 400(*)	P	86 g	+330 ml	2.5	400	1.84	11.5	57.5	15.7	10.86	11.96	4.68	6.47	2.57	0.07	0.06	9.41
Peptide formulae																		
MCP Pharm.	Salvipeptid	P	129 g	+400 ml	2.0	500	2.67	16.7	95.0	6.0	30.00	15.00	5.00	7.00	2.70	0.05	0.04	15.00
Merck	Peptisorbon	P	83 g	+400 ml	2.5	333	2.40	15.0	58.3	4.5	20.00	10.00	4.17	6.47	2.75	0.05	0.03	13.36
Roussel	Nutranel	P	101 g	+350 ml	2.8	396	2.52	15.8	74.3	4.0	8.00	14.20	4.60	4.64	1.64	0.07	0.04	9.60
Scientific	Pepdite 2†	P	100 g	+400 ml	2.0	450	2.22	13.9	63.0	18.1	9.13	13.20	5.00	6.79	2.93	0.08	0.07	4.80
Hospital Supplies	MCT Pepdite 2†*	P	100 g	+400 ml	2.0	460	2.22	13.9	62.4	18.8	13.47	13.20	5.00	6.79	2.93	0.08	0.07	4.80
Elemental formulae																		
Bristol-Myers	Flexical°	P	454 g	see instr.	0.5	2002	7.18	44.9	305.5	68.0	30.39	64.12	30.00	32.27	16.66	0.32	3.05	56.29
Norwich-Eaton	Vivonex – Standard*	P	80 g	+300 ml	3.3	300	0.97	6.2	69.0	0.4	11.21	9.01	4.16	5.33	2.73	0.05	0.03	15.40
Labs	– HN*	P	80 g	+300 ml	3.3	300	2.00	13.3	63.3	0.2	10.05	5.39	2.50	3.20	1.64	0.03	0.02	15.60
Scientific Hospital Supplies	Elemental 028*	P	100 g	+650 ml	1.3	400	1.92	10.0	77.8	6.6	10.86	11.94	4.68	6.47	2.57	0.07	0.06	9.40

1 Normal dilution for patients already established on a specific regimen. This may need to be modified when commencing a regimen. (Normal dilution made up with water according to manufacturer's recommendations).
2 Available in different size packages
3 State: L – Liquid presentation
   P – Powder presentation
* Lactose free formula   *MCT based formula   † Contains fibre

4 Tube feeding solutions: details of manufacturers

Manufacturer	*Product*
Abbott Laboratories Ltd.	Enrich
Queenborough	Ensure – Standard
Kent ME11 5EL	– Plus
Tel: 0795–663371	Osmolite
Bristol Myers Pharmaceuticals	Flexical
Station Road	
Langley	
Slough SL3 6EB	Isocal
Tel: Slough 44266	
Cow and Gate Limited	Fortison – Standard
Clinical Products Division,	– Energy Plus
PO Box 99	– Low Sodium
Trowbridge	– Soya
Wiltshire BA14 8YQ	Pre – Fortison
Tel: 02214–68381	
KabiVitrum Ltd.	Nutrauxil
KabiVitrum House	
Riverside Way	
Uxbridge	
Middlesex UB8 2YF	
Tel: 0895–51144	
MCP Pharmaceuticals Ltd.,	Salvimulsin MCT
Simpson Parkway,	
Kirkton Campus	Salvipeptid
Livingstone	
West Lothian EH54 7BH	
Tel: 0506–412512	
E. Merck Ltd.,	Peptisorbon
Winchester Road,	
Four Marks	Triosorbon
Alton	
Hampshire GU34 5HG	
Tel: 0420–64011	
Norwich-Eaton Pharmaceuticals	Vivonex-Standard
Regent House,	–HN
The Broadway,	
Woking,	
Surrey GU21 5AP	
Tel: 04862–71671	

Oxford Nutrition Ltd.,   Hipernutril MCT
PO Box 31   Stressnutril
Oxford OX2 8HB
Tel: 0865-58045

Roussel Laboratories Ltd.   Clinifeed – Iso
Broadwater Park,   – 400
North Orbital Road,   – Favour
Uxbridge   – Protein Rich
Middlesex UB9 5HP
Tel: 0895-834343   Nutranel

Scientific Hospital Supplies Ltd.,   Enteral 400
38, Queensland Street,   Pepdite
Liverpool L7 3JG   Elemental 028
Tel: 051-708-8008

Appendix VI

1 Nasogastric feeding
Intubation

Requirements: Gauze swabs
Nasogastric tube size 8 or finer (check length, etc.
and refrigerate for 5 minutes beforehand if
necessary)
Water and glass (ice cubes if preferred)
Gallipot × 2
Measuring jug
Kidney dish
2 ml syringe
Litmus paper
Universal container
$\frac{1}{2}$ inch Sterifix
Spigot (if necessary)

Procedure

1   Explain the procedure to the patient, draw the curtains and
bring the equipment.

2   Ensure the nostrils are clean.

3   Place the patient in a suitable comfortable position –
preferably sitting up.

4   Measure approximate length of tube required:

Nose to ear.
Ear to diaphragm.
Add these together to give an indication of the required length.

5   Lubricate tip of tube with water and insert the tube into the
nostril. It should be passed gently in a backward and downward
direction. Some tubes have special coatings which become slippery
when moistened with water.

NB   If an introducer is necessary the tube should only be
introduced by a qualified member of the medical staff.

6   Instruct the patient to swallow while the tube is being passed.
Sips of water or cubes of ice to suck may be given if fasting is not
essential. Observe the patient's colour throughout the procedure
and if he becomes cyanosed, withdraw the tube.

7   Pass tube until appropriate length indicator is against nostril.

8   To ensure that the tube is in the stomach:

a   Test gastric juice with litmus – attach syringe to tube and apply *gentle* suction until aspirate is obtained. This should show an acid reaction, i.e. blue litmus turns red.

b   Inject air via syringe down nasogastric tube. Listen with a stethoscope and this should elicit air sounds in the stomach.

c   X-ray – this is the preferred method when a fine bore tube is inserted.

These tests should be checked by a trained member of the nursing staff.

9   The tube should be spigotted. Attach the tube to the patient's nostril with Sterifix. The dressing should be *small* and unobtrusive.

10   Measure and record the amount and type of fluid aspirated.

11   If a specimen is required for laboratory tests, it should be put directly into the universal container from the first sample aspirated. Complete the label and send the specimen to the laboratory with the appropriate request form. It may be necessary to save a specimen of aspirate for the doctor to inspect.

12   Commence feeding according to the prescribed regimen.

2 Nasogastric feeding
Bolus feeding

Requirements: Tray
                   Feeding funnel, tubing and connection
                   Spigot
                   Gallipot × 2
                   Measuring jug
                   20 ml syringe (2 ml if fine bore tube used)
                   Litmus paper
                   Plain water
                   Paper towel
                   Prepared feeding solution
                   Water and syringe

Procedure

1 Wash hands.

2 Check name of patient and date of feed on container in refrigerator or on can/bottle (which does not require refrigeration).

3 Measure required amount of feed into a jug, and heat by standing jug in a bowl of hot water from the urn (the temperature should be 37–40°C).

4 Explain the procedure to the patient. Bring the equipment and draw the curtains.

5 Place the patient in the appropriate position; this is usually the upright position for the conscious patient and the lateral position for the unconscious patient, unless contra-indicated.

6 Wash hands.

7 Protect patient with paper towel, remove spigot from the nasogastric tube and place in gallipot.

8 Aspirate a sample of gastric contents with the syringe and test for acidity. This should be checked by a trained member of staff. Flush tube through with water. State amount used and enter on fluid chart.

9 Compress tubing attached to funnel, fill funnel with feed at correct temperature then with tubing compressed connect to nasogastric tube and run feed in slowly. (Do not hold the funnel too

high – this will cause the solution to be presented to the gut too quickly.) Avoid entry of air by keeping funnel refilled. Patient should be observed carefully throughout the procedure.

10   Finally give a measured amount of plain water to clean the nasogastric tube and enter this amount on fluid chart.

11   Disconnect funnel and tubing, replace spigot.

12   Record type and amount of feed on fluid balance chart together with any extra liquid used for flushing.

13   Clear away equipment, wash funnel and tubing through with 10 % Milton in the kitchen and leave inverted in clean, covered container.

14   If any feeding solution is left in the can/bottle make sure that this is appropriately covered and refrigerated to avoid bacterial proliferation.

15   Replace tray on locker, covered and ready for use.

3   Nasogastric feeding
    Continuous gravity drip feeding
    and pump assisted feeding

Requirements: Feeding solution
Giving set (it is necessary to use a giving set which
incorporates a silastic insert if an enteral feeding
pump is to be used)
Reservoir (some giving sets have an integral
reservoir)
Enteral feeding pump (if required)
Spigot (if necessary)

Procedure
  1   Wash hands.

  2   Explain the procedure to the patient, draw the curtains and
bring the equipment.

  3   Check the feeding solution is that which has been prescribed
for the patient.
The solution will be either:

a   Ready to administer in a sterile reservoir.

b   Presented in cans which may require dilution with water before
administration. Follow the instructions from Dietitian and ensure
that the contents are thoroughly mixed to avoid sedimentation.

c   Ready to administer 'home-made' feed, presented in plastic
cartons.

NB   *Do not use feeds for any patient other than the one for whom it is
intended.*
  4   Ensure that the nasogastric tube is in the correct position – see
procedure on intubation (p. 188).

  5   Attach the giving set to the reservoir if this is appropriate and
ensure the flow regulator is closed.

  6   Prime the drip chamber and run solution through giving set,
ensuring that all air is expelled from line.

  7   Attach the giving set to nasogastric tube.

  8   Adjust the clamp to give the required drip rate. Check the rate

after the first ten minutes and continue to monitor throughout the feeding period.

NB When using an enteral feeding pump, insert silastic section of the giving set into the machine and set rate to administer a continuous flow.

9 When the solution has been administered, remove giving set and reservoir and clear the nasogastric tube with 20−30 ml water and the spigot if necessary.

NB The giving set and reservoir should not be used for more than 24 hours without re-sterilisation.

10 Record type and amount of feed given and how much is left on the feeding chart and fluid balance chart, together with any extra liquid used for flushing.

11 If the reservoir is to be re-used, it should be thoroughly washed with an appropriate anionic detergent to remove all traces of feeding solution. The reservoir should then be filled with and completely immersed in 10 % Milton solution in a clean covered container. It is important that all equipment remains immersed until it is next required. Do not rinse before refilling with feed.

Appendix VII

1 Ranges of usual daily nutrient requirements for parenteral feeding

Nitrogen	8 – 20 g
Energy	1500 – 3000 kcal
Electrolytes and trace elements:	
Sodium	70 – 220 mmol
Potassium	60 – 120 mmol
Chloride	70 – 220 mmol
Calcium	5 – 10 mmol
Magnesium	5 – 20 mmol
Phosphate	20 – 40 mmol
Zinc	2 – 7 mg
Copper	1.6 mg
Selenium	120 μg
Iodine	120 μg
Chromium (trivalent)	50 μg
Vitamins	
A	5700 iu
B_1	28.6 mg
B_2	5.7 mg
Nicotinamide	57 mg
Pantothenate	14.3 mg
B_6	8.6 mg
C	286 mg
E	2.9 mg
Folic acid	15 mg per week
K_1	10 mg per month
B_{12}	250 μg per 2 months

2. Some available intravenous amino acid solutions: composition per litre

	Non-protein Calories	Nitrogen g	Na mmol	K mmol	Mg mmol	PO_4 mmol	Ca mmol	Cl mmol
Vamin N	—	9.4	50	20	1.5	—	2.5	55
Vamin Glucose	400	9.4	50	20	1.5	—	2.5	55
Vamin 14	—	13.5	100	50	8.0	—	5.0	100
Aminoplex 14	—	13.4	35	30	—	—	—	79
Vamin 14 (no electrolytes)	—	13.5	—	—	—	—	—	—
Freamine II	—	12.5	10	—	—	10	—	—
Synthamin 9	—	9.3	73	60	5.0	30	—	70
Vamin 18 (no electrolytes)	—	18.0	—	—	—	—	—	—
Synthamin 14	—	14.3	73	60	5.0	30	—	70

Some available intravenous calorie solutions

	Non-protein Calories	Nitrogen g	Na mmol	K mmol	Mg mmol	PO_4 mmol	Ca mmol	Cl mmol
Dextrose 20%	760	—	—	—	—	—	—	—
Dextrose A (20%)	760	—	—	—	28.0	—	26.0	—
Dextrose B (20%)	760	—	—	60	—	60	—	—
Intralipid 10%	1000	—	—	—	—	15	—	—
Intralipid 20%	2000	—	—	—	—	15	—	—

NB For 10 g of nitrogen and 2000 calories relative cost compared to cheapest enteral feeding = £30 more

3. Vitamin solutions for intravenous infusion

	Recommended daily intake	Multibionta	Parentrovite IVHP ampoule 1	Parentrovite IVHP ampoule 2	Solivito	Vitlipid Adult	Intralipid 20% (500 ml)
Thiamine (mg) B$_1$	1.4	50	250	—	1.2	—	—
Riboflavin (mg) B$_2$	2.1	7.29	4.0	—	1.8	—	—
Pyridoxine (mg) B$_6$	2.1	15	50	—	2.0	—	—
Cyanocobalamin (µg) B$_{12}$	2.0	—	—	—	2.0	—	—
Nicotinamide (mg)	14	100	—	160	10	—	—
Biotin (mg)	0.35	—	—	—	0.3	—	—
Pantothenic acid/dexpanthenol (mg)	14	25	—	—	10	—	—
Folic acid (mg)	2	—	—	—	0.2	—	—
Ascorbic acid (mg) VITC	35	500	—	500	30	—	—
Calciferol (IU) VITD	100	—	—	—	—	120	—
Phytylmenaquinone (µg)	140	—	—	—	—	150	—
Retinol (IU)	700	10000	—	—	—	2500	—
Tocopheryl acetate (IU)	30	5	—	—	—	—	30

4. Daily electrolyte and trace element requirements for intravenous feeding and solutions available: contents per litre

	Na^+ (mmol)	K^+ (mmol)	Mg^+ (mmol)	Ca^{2+} (mmol)	Zn^{2+} (μmol)	Mn^{2+} (μmol)	Fe^{3+} (μmol)	Cu^{2+} (μmol)	Cl^- (mmol)	PO_4^{3-} (mmol)	F^- (μmol)	I^- (μmol)
Recommended daily requirement	70–220	60–120	5–20	5–10	50	7	70	5	70–220	20–40	50	1
Addamel (Kabivitrum) per 10 ml ampoule	—	—	1.5	5	20	40	50	5	13	—	50	1
Electrolyte A (Travenol)	—	—	28	26	80	40	—	—	108	—	—	—
Electrolyte B (Travenol)	—	60	—	—	—	—	—	—	—	60	—	—
Glucoplex 1600 (Geistlich)	50	30	3	—	46	—	—	—	67	18	—	—

Appendix VIII

1 Introduction to intravenous nursing procedures

The aim of nursing management is to maintain catheter security and patency, and prevent infection. Success depends on rigorous adherence to established protocol, although this may be influenced by the site of catheter insertion, for example those inserted into the jugular vein or arm veins are readily kinked by patient movement. Tunnelling the catheter through the subcutaneous tissues, away from the site of venous insertion, to emerge at a flat area, usually on the anterior chest wall, increases the effectiveness of nursing care by allowing dressings to be maintained more easily and preventing the catheter being dislodged or kinked.

The catheter may be accidentally moved or pulled out if the sutures securing it become loose. Special precautions are needed with 'through needle' catheters to ensure that the needle guard remains firmly closed, thus preventing the catheter being cut and air entering the circulation as catheter embolism.

Another aspect of catheter security concerns the elimination of air from any part of the infusion system. Non-vented containers, Luer locks on administration sets and proper taping of connections to prevent traction, are important safeguards. Negative intra-thoracic pressure during inspiration may draw air into the circulation during the daily changing of administration set unless the patient is positioned flat and asked to perform the valsalva manoeuvre, straining against a closed glottis, or the catheter is first clamped. However, frequent clamping may fracture the catheter; therefore, a short extension tube may be interposed between the catheter and administration set for clamping purposes, this tube being changed weekly. The clamp should always be immediately to hand in case of accidental disconnection.

2 Central venous catheterisation

Ideally this should be performed in the operating theatre. Patients should be prepared as for theatre and male patients have the upper chest shaved on both sides to the level of the nipple. Catheterisation is performed under local anaesthetic and, unless contra-indicated, fluids may be taken freely during the preceding hours; however, food intake should be limited as the patient will be required to lie with the head tipped down and a full stomach can cause discomfort.

Pethidine and diazepam will be given intravenously immediately prior to the procedure; therefore, analgesia may not need to be given in the ward. Following the catheterisation, observe the patient for dyspnoea, pain in the chest, back or shoulders, or restlessness, and notify medical staff immediately should these symptoms occur.

The catheter will be tunnelled through the subcutaneous tissues and the primary insertion sutures at the clavicle should be removed after one week.

A chest X-ray to confirm the position of the catheter will be performed before the patient returns to the ward.

3 Problem solving

Infusion stopped
a Check for any twists or kinks in catheter or administration set.
b Close flow control valve. Release and open valve.
c Flush catheter. **NB** Not to be performed by inexperienced staff.

Equipment
5 ml Hepsal
Prescription sheet
2 ml syringe
Filter straw
5 sterile gauze squares
2 sterile towels
Sterile gloves
Chlorhexidine in spirit
Masks
Clamps

Procedure
Wash trolley, spray with spirit. Allow 2 minutes drying time.

Patient and nurse put on masks. Wash hands.

Place Hepsal at one side of trolley top. Spray with spirit.

Open one sterile towel across other side of trolley; onto it, open syringe filter straw, gauze and gloves.

Spray connection between extension tube and catheter; place a sterile towel under it.

Spray clamp and attach to catheter.

Put on gloves. Holding Hepsal in gauze square snap off top and draw up through filter straw. Connect filter straw to syringe.

Disconnect extension tube from catheter. Insert hub of syringe. (Place end of extension tube in gauze.)

Remove clamp.

Irrigate the catheter *allowing the pressure to build up gradually to avoid splitting the catheter.*

Clamp catheter.

Reconnect extension tube, remove clamp and regulate flow.

NB If catheter is still blocked, notify member of medical staff immediately.

Catheter fracture
Clamp catheter distal to fracture. Wrap spirit-soaked gauze around fracture and notify member of medical staff immediately.

Accidental disconnection of infusion system
Immediately place clamp distal to the disconnection. Use new giving set and container to recommence infusion.

Disconnection followed by faintness and breathlessness
Clamp system as above. Lie patient flat with feet elevated and call urgent medical help.

Damage to fluid container or next container unavailable
Continue infusion with dextrose 10 % at the rate prescribed for nutrient solution. Get advice from pharmacy.

Hypoglycaemia – dizziness, irritability, palpitations, excessive sweating
Check that the rate of flow has not been reduced from that prescribed and reset if necessary. If patient is able to take fluids give glucose drinks.

Hyperglycaemia – drowsiness, excessive urine output compared to fluid intake, sugar in the urine
Check that the rate of flow has not exceeded that prescribed. Call medical help.

4   Dressing change at TPN catheter site

Equipment used:
Chlorhexidine 0.5 w/v in spirit 70 %
Povidone Iodine Dry Spray Powder
Op-site spray dressing
Mepore dressing

Trolley
Dressing pack
Pair of sterile gloves
Mepore dressing
Chlorhexidine 0.5 % in spirit 70 %
Povidone iodine spray
Op-site spray
Tape

Patient and nurses put on masks.

Wash hands, wash trolley and spray with spirit – allow 2 minutes drying time.

Open out dressing pack. Pour Chlorhexidine/spirit into gallipot.

Open sterile gloves and Mepore dressing onto sterile field.

Loosen old dressing. Wash hands.

Lift off old dressing with one pair of forceps. Discard forceps and dressing. Inspect for redness or discharge – take swab if necessary.

Swab around insertion site with Chlorhexidine/spirit (from insertion point outwards).

Spray with povidone iodine.

Spray with Op-site.

Put on sterile gloves and apply Mepore dressing.

Tape up catheter to dressing and date.

5   Starting a TPN infusion

When it is possible for the Pharmacy department to provide them, three litre bags, containing nutritional requirements for 24 hours, should be used. These have the advantage of reducing the nursing time required for frequent bottle changes and the possibility of contamination. Special attention must be paid to the rate of administration which, if exceeded, may result in the patient receiving a large volume of hypertonic solution in a short period of time.

To change a three litre bag:

Equipment:
　Three litre bag and prescription sheet
　Two sterile dressing towels
　Sterile gloves
　New giving set
　Chlorhexidine 0.5 % in spirit 70 %
　Masks
　Clamp

Patient and nurse put on masks.

Wash hands, wash trolley and spray with spirit. Allow 2 minutes drying time.

Check three litre bag. Hang it up and remove blue cap. Spray around the lower half of bag.

NB   Requires two minutes drying time to achieve full effect.

Open out one sterile towel, place across patient's upper abdomen.

Spray connection between old giving set and extension tube and without touching sprayed area lay it across sterile towel.

Open out second sterile towel onto top of trolley. Onto it open new giving set and sterile gloves.

Apply clamp to upper part of extension tube. Close valve on old giving set.

Put on gloves. Insert new giving set into bag. Run fluid through.

Disconnect old set and connect new one.

Remove clamp and regulate flow.

To change extension tube:
Spray connection between catheter and extension tube and clamp catheter.

Connect new tube to new giving set. Run fluid through.

Disconnect extension tube from catheter and connect new one.

6   To use a volumetric infusion pump

Trolley
   Three litre bag and prescription chart
   Two sterile towels
   Pair of sterile gloves
   Appropriate giving set
   Chlorhexidine 0.5 % in spirit 70 % spray
   Masks
   Clamp

Wash trolley, spray with spirit. Allow 2 minutes drying time.
Wash hands.
Patient and nurses put on masks.

1st Nurse	*2nd Nurse*
Hang up bag, remove blue cap and spray around the lower half of bag.	
Open out sterile towel onto top of trolley. Onto it open giving set and gloves. Open second sterile towel across patient's upper abdomen and spray connection between extension tube and giving set.	Switch off pump.
Put on gloves. Tighten connections at either side of giving set.	Clamp extension tube. Remove old cassette from pump. Set volume and rate to 0.
Insert giving set into bag. Hand cassette to second nurse keeping hold of distal end.	Insert new cassette. Switch on pump and press purge button to expel air. Tap air out of the two injection ports.
When the set is free from air disconnect old giving set from extension tube and reconnect new one.	Switch off pump.
Remove clamp. Push tubing into air sensor.	
Set rate and volume to be infused and switch on.	

7 Changing giving set for two bottle system

Equipment:
 Bottles and prescription sheet
 Bottle hanger
 New giving set
 Airway if required
 Two sterile towels
 Sterile gloves
 Chlorhexidine 0.5 % in spirit 70 %
 Masks
 Clamp

Patient and nurse put on masks.

Wash hands. Wash trolley. Spray trolley with spirit. Allow 2 minutes drying time.

Check bottles. Stand them to one side of trolley top. Remove protective cap and spray with spirit.

Open out sterile towel across patient's upper abdomen. Spray connection between old giving set and extension tube. Without touching sprayed area lay it across sterile towel.

Open second sterile towel onto trolley top. Open giving set, airways and gloves onto it.

Apply clamp to upper part of extension tube. Close flow valve on old giving set.

Put on one sterile glove. Handling sterile equipment with gloved hand and holding bottle with ungloved hand insert new giving set and airway and hang bottles.

Put on other sterile glove. Run fluid through the set. Disconnect old giving set and connect new one.

Remove clamp and regulate flow.

8 Changing bottles

Equipment:
New bottles and prescription sheet
Sterile towel
Airway if required
Sterile gloves
Masks
Clamp
Chlorhexidine 0.5 % in spirit 70 %

Nurse puts on mask.

Wash hands, wash trolley, spray with spirit. Allow 2 minutes drying time.

Spray empty bottle and connection between it and giving set.

Check new bottle, stand it to one side of trolley top. Remove protective cap and spray.

Onto other side of trolley open sterile towel, onto it open an airway if required and sterile gloves.

Close flow valve. Put on sterile gloves. Insert airway. Remove giving set from empty bottle and insert new one. Hang bottle and regulate flow.

9 Heparinising Catheter

Equipment:
  Hepsal.
  Prescription sheet
  5 ml syringe
  Filter straw
  Orange needle
  Luer spigot
  Sterile gloves
  2 sterile towels
  Sterile gauze squares
  Clamp
  Masks
  Chlorhexidine 0.5 % in spirit 70 %

Patient and nurse put on masks.

Wash hands, wash trolley and spray with spirit. Allow 2 minutes drying time.

Place Hepsal to one side of trolley top and spray.

Open out one sterile towel onto other side of trolley top. Onto it open syringe, filter straw, orange needle, Luer locking spigot, gauze and gloves.

Open second sterile towel across patient's upper abdomen. Spray connection between extension tube and giving set. Without touching sprayed area lay it across sterile towel. Apply clamp to upper part of extension tube. Close flow valve on giving set.

Put on sterile gloves. Connect filter straw to syringe. Holding the Hepsal in one gauze square, snap top and draw up after checking dose.

Change filter straw for orange needle.

Disconnect giving set from extension tube. Connect Luer spigot.

Insert needle through diaphragm of spigot. Release clamp. Withdraw air bubble. Without disconnecting syringe allow it to float to top of fluid in the syringe. Inject Hepsal.

10   Removal of tunnelled central venous catheter

Equipment:
Dressing pack including sterile scissors
Stitch cutter
Sterile occlusive elastoplast dressing
Chlorhexidine 0.5 % in spirit 70 %
Sterile specimen jar
Masks

Patient and nurse put on masks.

Wash hands, wash trolley and spray with spirit. Allow 2 minutes drying time.

Open dressing pack. Pour out Chlorhexidine in spirit. Onto sterile field, open elastoplast dressing and stitch cutter.

Remove old dressing.

Clean around insertion site with Chlorhexidine in spirit and remove sutures.

Place a cotton wool ball soaked in spirit solution above insertion site.

Remove lid from specimen jar.

Withdraw catheter, allowing spirit-soaked swab to fall over skin puncture.

Take the sterile scissors from the dressing pack and cut the tip from the catheter allowing it to fall directly into the specimen jar. Replace the lid on the jar.

Apply sterile elastoplast to puncture site.

Send catheter tip labelled with form to Bacteriology.

NB   Broviac catheters must be removed by a member of the medical staff.

11   Peripheral vein cannula insertion

This is an aseptic procedure.

Trolley:
  Dressing pack
  Clinical sheets
  Sterile gloves
  Chlorhexidine 0.5% in spirit 70%
  Povidone iodine spray
  (local anaesthetic if desired, 5 ml syringe and orange needle)
  Cannula of choice
  Extension tube
  Luer-locking spigot
  Hepsal 2 ml syringe, filter straw and orange needle
  Steri-Strips (sterile)
  Razor
  Mepore dressing

Wash hands well.

Shave patient's skin gently if necessary.

Clean the arm with chlorhexidine 0.5% in spirit 70%.

Allow to dry, then spray with povidone iodine.

Put on sterile gloves.

Use local anaesthetic if desired.

Prepare injection of 2 ml Hepsal, attach orange needle.

Connect Luer-locking spigot to extension tube.

Pierce the latex cap of the spigot with the orange needle and fill the tube with Hepsal. Insert cannula.

When the cannula is in position connect the extension tube and complete the injection of Hepsal.

Clean the povidone iodine powder off the skin with spirit.

Allow to dry, then tape the cannula with sterile Steri-Strips (these will not stick over iodine powder).

Spray povidone iodine over puncture site.

Apply Mepore dressing.

Do not apply any further bandages or splints.

Procedure for cannula removal:
Remove the tape.

Clean skin with chlorhexidine 0.5 % in spirit 70 %; allow to dry.
Withdraw cannula, cut off end into sterile container using sterile scissors.

Label and send to Bacteriology immediately.

Appendix IX

1 Commonly encountered complications during nutrition and their correction

Complication	Clinical Presentation	Cause	Correction
Low serum sodium	Confusion Apathy	Water intoxication GI or renal loss	Reduce water intake Increase Na^+ intake
Low serum potassium	Apathy Cardiac irregularity	Inadequate K^+ intake GI or renal loss	Increase K^+ intake
Low serum magnesium	Weakness Vertigo Convulsions	Inadequate Mg^{2+} intake GI or renal loss	Increase Mg^{2+}
Low serum phosphate	Apathy, confusion, Paralysis, RBC Oxygen dissociation	Inadequate inorganic phosphate intake	Increase PO_4 intake
High blood sugar	Increased blood sugar	Unsuspected diabetes Underlying sepsis Excess infusion of carbohydrate (IV)	Treat underlying cause Treat underlying cause Reduce infusion rate (IV)
Low blood sugar	Lethargy	Interrupted infusion	Give dextrose

2 Monitoring feeding regimens

Daily

Body weight
Fluid balance
Full blood count, urea & electrolytes
Blood glucose
Electrolyte & nitrogen analysis of urine & gastro-intestinal losses
Acid base status

Three Times Weekly

Serum calcium, magnesium & phosphate
Plasma proteins
Liver function tests
Clotting studies

Ten Days

Serum B_{12}, folate, haemoglobin, iron, lactate & triglycerides
Trace elements including zinc

Index